Becoming a Midwife

A Student Guide

T0347726

Study Skills

Academic Success
Academic Writing Skills for International Students
Ace Your Exam
Becoming a Critical Thinker
Be Well, Learn Well
Brilliant Essays
The Business Student's Phrase Book
Cite Them Right (12th edn)
Critical Thinking and Persuasive Writing for Postgraduates
Critical Thinking for Nursing, Health and Social Care
Critical Thinking Skills (3rd edn)
Dissertations and Project Reports
Doing Projects and Reports in Engineering
The Employability Journal
Essentials of Essay Writing
The Exam Skills Handbook (2nd edn)
Get Sorted
The Graduate Career Guidebook (2nd edn)
Great Ways to Learn Anatomy and Physiology (2nd edn)
How to Use Your Reading in Your Essays (3rd edn)
How to Write Better Essays (5th edn)
How to Write Your Literature Review
How to Write Your Undergraduate Dissertation (3rd edn)
Improve Your Grammar (3rd edn)
The Bloomsbury Student Planner
Mindfulness for Students
Presentation Skills for Students (3rd edn)
The Principles of Writing in Psychology
Professional Writing (4th edn)
Reading at University
Reflective Writing for Nursing, Health and Social Work
Simplify Your Study
Skills for Business and Management
Skills for Success (4th edn)
Stand Out from the Crowd
The Student Phrase Book (2nd edn)
The Student's Guide to Writing (3rd edn)
The Study Skills Handbook (5th edn)
Study Skills for International Postgraduates (2nd edn)
Studying in English
Studying Law (4th edn)
The Study Success Journal
Success in Academic Writing (2nd edn)
Smart Thinking
Teaching Study Skills and Supporting Learning
The Undergraduate Research Handbook (2nd edn)
The Work-Based Learning Student Handbook (3rd edn)
Writing for Biomedical Sciences Students
Writing for Engineers (4th edn)
Writing for Nursing and Midwifery Students (3rd edn)

Write it Right (2nd edn)
Writing for Science Students (2nd edn)
Writing Skills for Education Students
Writing Skills for Social Work Students
You2Uni: Decide, Prepare, Apply

Pocket Study Skills

14 Days to Exam Success (2nd edn)
Analyzing a Case Study
Brilliant Writing Tips for Students
Completing Your PhD
Doing Research (2nd edn)
Getting Critical (3rd edn)
How to Analyze Data
Managing Stress
Planning Your Dissertation (2nd edn)
Planning Your Essay (3rd edn)
Planning Your PhD
Posters and Presentations
Reading and Making Notes (3rd edn)
Referencing and Understanding Plagiarism (2nd edn)
Reflective Writing (2nd edn)
Report Writing (2nd edn)
Science Study Skills
Studying with Dyslexia (2nd edn)
Success in Groupwork (2nd edn)
Successful Applications
Time Management
Using Feedback to Boost Your Grades
Where's Your Argument? (2nd edn)
Where's Your Evidence?
Writing for University (3rd edn)

50 Ways

50 Ways to Boost Your Grades
50 Ways to Boost Your Employability
50 Ways to Excel at Writing
50 Ways to Manage Stress
50 Ways to Manage Time Effectively
50 Ways to Succeed as an International Student

Research Skills

Authoring a PhD
The Foundations of Research (3rd edn)
Getting to Grips with Doctoral Research
Getting Published
The Good Supervisor (2nd edn)
The Lean PhD
Maximizing the Impacts of Academic Research
PhD by Published Work
The PhD Viva
The PhD Writing Handbook
Planning Your Postgraduate Research
The Postgraduate's Guide to Research Ethics
The Postgraduate Research Handbook (2nd edn)
The Professional Doctorate
Structuring Your Research Thesis

Becoming a Midwife

A Student Guide

Ellie Durant

BLOOMSBURY ACADEMIC
LONDON • NEW YORK • OXFORD • NEW DELHI • SYDNEY

BLOOMSBURY ACADEMIC
Bloomsbury Publishing Plc
50 Bedford Square, London, WC1B 3DP, UK
1385 Broadway, New York, NY 10018, USA
29 Earlsfort Terrace, Dublin 2, Ireland

BLOOMSBURY, BLOOMSBURY ACADEMIC and the Diana logo
are trademarks of Bloomsbury Publishing Plc

First published in Great Britain 2023

A catalogue record for this book is available from the British Library.

Library of Congress Cataloging-in-Publication Data
Names: Durant, Ellie, author.
Title: Becoming a midwife : a student guide / Ellie Durant.
Description: London ; New York : Bloomsbury Academic, 2023. |
Series: Bloomsbury study skills | Includes bibliographical references and index. |
Summary: "Written in a friendly, uplifting tone, Becoming a Midwife : A Student Guide provides
students and newly-qualified midwives with the tools and support they need to thrive on their
course, on placement and in the early stages of their careers.
Chapters are enriched with insights from students and practising midwives,
practical tips, worksheets to promote reflective practice and suggestions for further reading.
Covering core academic skills, the fundamentals of clinical practice, self-care and the transition
to newly-qualified midwife, this is the go-to guide to help student midwifes not only
survive but thrive on their course" – Provided by publisher.
Identifiers: LCCN 2022032119 (print) | LCCN 2022032120 (ebook) |
ISBN 9781350322332 (paperback) | ISBN 9781350322349 (pdf) |
ISBN 9781350322356 (epub) | ISBN 9781350322363
Subjects: LCSH: Midwifery.
Classification: LCC RG950 .D87 2023 (print) | LCC RG950
(ebook) | DDC 618.2–dc23/eng/20220719
LC record available at https://lccn.loc.gov/2022032119
LC ebook record available at https://lccn.loc.gov/2022032120

ISBN: PB: 978-1-3503-2233-2
          ePDF: 978-1-3503-2234-9
          eBook: 978-1-3503-2235-6

Series: Bloomsbury Study Skills

Typeset by Integra Software Services Pvt. Ltd.

To find out more about our authors and books visit www.bloomsbury.com
and sign up for our newsletters.

Contents

To the students and midwives who keep turning up and making a difference.

Introduction

I'd like to start this book with a quote from a blog post I wrote about my early training:

> ... you get told a lot that 'you're at university level now, you won't be spoon fed', 'you need to develop rhino skin', etc. At the time I thought I hadn't experienced enough of life to be good at absorbing criticism. The reality of the situation looking back on it is that being on a midwifery degree involves more feedback and constructive criticism than most other adult settings ... I've come to realise that when people look good at learning, it's because they have a bedrock of self-belief. The task, which is a brave one, is to find some support and self-worth and to feel like we deserve that. We have to find ways of building ourselves up rather than tearing ourselves down.

Midwifery has a high student attrition rate. In the UK, which is where I'm based, we lose about 30 per cent of midwifery students before qualification (though 8.5 per cent of these have an interruption of their studies and go on to complete at a later date) (Astrup 2018). The Royal College of Midwives cites evidence that 5 to 10 per cent of newly qualified midwives in the UK leave in their first year and 50 per cent of midwives in their first five years of practice are considering leaving (RCM 2020: 4). In 2017 I ran a conference addressing the culture of midwifery that focused on bullying and how to prevent it. I'm not denying the problems in midwifery, there are many, and I'm clearly not immune to them.

However, even when I took a break from clinical midwifery for medical reasons I was still captivated by the profession and started a blog and Facebook community to support student and newly qualified midwives. I rejoined the register in 2021 and at the time of writing, I am still glowing from one beautiful birth on New Year's Eve and another in early 2022. Sometimes I can't believe how lucky I am to be invited to be involved in these births. Midwifery is a paradox: it has brought me to my knees and also made me glad to be who I am. I think like many other people who sign up to study midwifery, I was aware that it was going to be more than I could handle on some days, but I also knew it would help me lead a meaningful life. It has delivered on those things.

Back when I was at the start of my degree I was missing some of the fundamental learning skills that would have made my training so much easier. There is a lot of assistance out there to guide you on your academic work and I hope I've charted some of these areas. I have covered academic skills around essays, exams and giving presentations, and the book then progresses to two midwifery theory skills which may be new to you: writing reflections and appraising research. I have also included lots of ideas for the practice part of your course, including the advocacy and activism skills that are so challenging, but so beneficial for both clients and midwives. I then cover job applications, a favourite topic of mine as doing well with this process can open doors for you, and the skills involved are attainable. Finally, I discuss what it feels like to be newly qualified and the practical elements needed to move into your new role.

It's important to point out that this book is about the things I wish I'd known before starting training as a midwife, supplemented with everything I've learnt over the last three-plus years of writing. Just like having a baby, you can listen to the 'experts', but only you will know how to tailor ideas to your particular needs and life. Don't feel you have to follow every suggestion, just take the techniques you think are useful, and make them your own.

Even when your training is difficult, I want you to know that your contribution is important and it's crucial to look after yourself as much as you can. This book is an attempt to help you work out where you fit and how you can give ongoing brilliant care to women and birthing people.

Thanks for choosing midwifery.

Eleanor (Ellie) Durant

Time Management

Introduction

Given the demands of midwifery training and everything you have to achieve, the number one thing you'll need to be good at (apart from being kind to the people around you) is time management. There are lots of time management ideas in this chapter that I wish I'd known before I started my midwifery degree. I'll share some ideas from students and midwives, and then explain a concept that will help you prioritize. Then I'll concentrate on a to-do list method that has some evidence behind it in terms of increasing positive outlook and self-belief (Allen 2015: 259; Heylighen and Vidal 2008). It's something I've used since I began to work on researching this book and has stood up to life on a return to practice course, and then as a practising midwife, all while simultaneously writing and running a business.

What I found in my research is that good time management comes down to being able to create islands of time in which to concentrate, even if you have a million different things on the horizon. Intuition is a big part of time management and only you know what will work for your personality.

Time management tips from students and midwives

Before we get on with the to-do list strategy, I wanted to share some techniques from students and midwives that were shared in the online community I run.

This last point in Box 1.1 is key. Midwifery is such a weighty job sometimes. You need that lightness, you can't walk around with the weight of the world on your shoulders all the time.

Watching me write those first few assignments must have been like watching someone trying to drink the ocean. My love of doing a deep dive into a topic has not disappeared, but these days I try to temper it with an idea known as 80/20, and it means I don't get overwhelmed as often.

Box 1.1: Time management tips from students and midwives

1. Get to know your process. Patterns of your best work will start to emerge. You might be an early morning person, you might need to do exercise first. You might need a chat with a good friend to get some things off your mind. You might work best for a few hours just as everyone else goes to sleep.

2. Don't compare yourself to anyone else, especially those you know only from social media. We only get snapshots of other people even in real life, and online it's even more difficult to know what's going on behind the scenes. We all have different skills and midwifery clients need that diversity from us, so comparing yourself to others is wasted energy.

3. Learn to say no. If there's something you don't really want to do, and it's not essential, politely decline. 'I'm afraid it's not a great time for me to do that' is my phrase.

4. Use only the correct amount of discipline for you. I often go to bed early, get up early and make sure I'm on task or a few hours before anyone else gets up. But if you push yourself too hard you can end up frustrated and with no energy.

    Take good lecture notes, bearing in mind what you will end up using them for. For content that will be useful when you're revising for an exam, bullet points, clear diagrams and detail are probably best. If the lecture covers topics you think might be useful when writing an assignment, you might include more abstract ideas or areas which you want to flag for further reading, and references are key.

5. On a basic life maintenance note, have your supermarket shop delivered if you can afford it. And batch cook. Pretty much every student midwife will tell you this.

    Make your own mind up about how hard the course is. Your experience of the work will depend on your previous academic background, life experience, support and so many other factors. Don't let people wind you up, training as a midwife is a lot like parenthood in that everyone wants to tell you their horror stories. But be open to the fact that it might turn out just fine.

6. You will put more energy into your degree and career if you have some fun with your friends at least once a week. Also, try to find some friends within midwifery; hopefully, people who can reframe midwifery challenges as funny.

80/20 – How to prioritize as a student midwife

The principle of 80/20 says that in many situations, 80 per cent of the output comes from 20 per cent of the input. The idea comes from a Victorian-era economist who noticed that in many countries, 80 per cent of the wealth was owned by 20 per cent of people. This idea spread because the 80/20 ratio seems to apply to lots of other disciplines; for instance, in biology often the top 20 per cent of plants are responsible for 80 per cent of reproduction (Marques 2021; Tanabe 2018). It's a consistent maths concept that you can apply to your own life. For example, I bet you wear about 20 per cent of your clothes 80 per cent of the time. 80/20 is currently a pop culture reference, you'll see it on business blogs, in YouTube videos and so on (Ferriss 2022). It's appealing because it says that in any given situation, 20 per cent of the actions you take will be responsible for 80 per cent of the results, which means you can skip a lot of work.

When I first came across 80/20 I was annoyed and thought it was cynical and couldn't apply to midwifery because everything we learn and do is so important. However, midwifery is a huge subject that traditionally pulls from many other disciplines like obstetrics, nursing, social work, psychology, etc. We have to find somewhere to start, some way of deciding what to focus on. The 80/20 rule should prompt you to ask 'What are the vital bits I need to pay attention to here? What are the sources I should read first?' Of course, another angle on all this is that 80/20 helps us cut through our perfectionism.

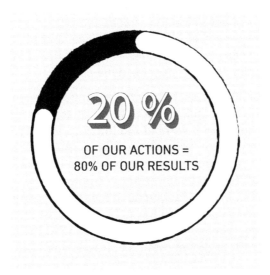

20 %
OF OUR ACTIONS =
80% OF OUR RESULTS

If you can get a handle on your work quickly by concentrating on the essentials, you'll have time left over for your passion projects. You can then apply much more effort in these vital areas.

Answering the question 'What is the top 20 per cent of the information I should be concentrating on here?' is hard. Don't beat yourself up if you're overwhelmed and can't seem to get 80/20 to work. If it's not for you, that's fine: I think my initial immersion into midwifery might have been an essential part of the process for me, and in many ways I wouldn't change it. But 80/20 can be a common-sense way of approaching what can seem an impossible task. It may be that 80/20 doesn't work for you in some cases, but in others it makes all the difference. It's now one of my tools for both clinical midwifery and academic learning.

My to-do list method

During a midwifery course you'll have significant information coming at you from family, friends, independent study, lectures, podcasts, WhatsApp groups, your practice supervisor, the student loan company, and so on. You'll have to balance the urgency of tasks that need doing now with those that need long-term tracking and time commitment. You'll also have a lot of unpredictability to contend with. You might have an essay due and so want to finish your shift on time but saying to a client, 'Sorry you had a huge bleed and your premature baby isn't very well but I'm off' isn't something student midwives find easy to do.

The to-do list method I use involves writing down everything I have to do and sorting it into tables with different useful headings. I find that once I've done this, prioritizing becomes easy as I can see what needs to be done at a glance. You can also take into account your fluctuating energy levels, and any extra time that appears because you have a slow day on placement, etc. The point is to get your tasks into a form that means you can use your gut feeling rather than complex calculations about what needs to be done next.

You will also be able to sort essential from non-essential tasks so you don't waste time, and renegotiate tasks so if plan A doesn't work you can find plan B without too much trouble. I find I also avoid that constant feeling of 'I should be doing something else'. This system takes a few hours to set up, but there is research evidence supporting this strategy in line with self-efficacy theory (Heylighen and Vidal 2008). Like any technique, it's hard to explain how well it works on paper. I suggest you try it. Take a look at the blank to-do list tables below (you can also jump to the end of the chapter to see a student midwife to-do list that has already been processed).

Table 1.1: Proforma to-do list

The In-List			
Urgent			
Exams	Begin with ...	Location	Defer until ...
Placement	Begin with ...	Location	Defer until ...
Assignments	Begin with ...	Location	Defer until ...
Family	Begin with ...	Location	Defer until ...
Someday/Maybe	Begin with ...	Location	Defer until ...

To fill in these tables you will need to ...

1. Capture

You'll need somewhere to write down everything in a big unprocessed to-do list. In *Getting Things Done* (Allen 2015), which is where I found this method, this is called 'The In List'. It should be a bit of a mess. The key thing is for you to capture every potential task you have to do, even if you're not sure if it's essential. This means you won't have missed any responsibilities or opportunities.

Back before technology took off, your capture method might have been a pocket notebook. These days what might be easier is a smartphone with a file on your home screen (something like Google Docs or Evernote) where you can record all the tasks you need to think about.

The point at this stage isn't to take action – it's to record absolutely everything as a matter of course so you can be confident about not forgetting anything. I find this useful as it means I have headspace because I know I've recorded everything important.

2. Process

You then will have to process all of the tasks you've written down. This means you give them consideration and put them into the right table in your document, meaning they can be dealt with at the right point in your life. There are three parts to processing an in list:

a. As you move through your list, first put anything that has a fixed time and date on your calendar. For instance, an assignment deadline or conference you're attending should go on your calendar asap.

b. Then sort things into subdivisions of lists. These are usually things like exams, assignments, placement, life admin, read/reference material list, someday/maybe and incubate. As mentioned, I use tables to do this.

   The best of this system is you can see instantly what you can do right now and what you need to know or wait for in order to complete any outstanding task. For instance, if you want to wait until you've been to a research critique seminar before starting your essay, you can put that date and detail in the 'defer until' column.

c. I process my in list when it gets long, which can be once every week or once a month depending on how busy I am. I will go through and delete things from my to-do list about every two months.

Box 1.2: Top tips

There are three more parts of this to-do list strategy.

1. I often colour code my tasks in terms of the location of that activity – library, home, hospital, etc. This makes it easy to batch tasks.

   Within reason, if something takes less than three minutes to do, do it there and then.

2. Don't put the things you want to get done on your calendar, it's just for fixed tasks or appointments. Otherwise, it can quickly become hard to pick out what's absolutely essential.

Adding assignments to your to-do list

Essays, assignments and exam revision are projects that might start off in a general 'assignments' list but will eventually graduate to having their own table.

For example, a specific table for an essay might look like the following.

Table 1.2: Essay project to-do list

Essay project	Begin with ...	Location	Defer until ...
	Write due date on calendar	home	
	Choose topic	library	First assignment submitted (10th sept)
	Plan research period and assign dates for this	home	
	Plans dates for writing and assign dates for this	home	
	Plan dates for reviewing/ submitting early to tutor for feedback/ assign dates for this	Ask at uni	Know dates of lectures with tutor

Box 1.3: Extra useful ideas for your to-do list

1. On my to-do list I keep a link to a 'reading/review' file. This is a Google document I have for when I come across an interesting article or resource but don't have time to read it right then. This file is great because if I'm delayed on a train or waiting for something, I can find something I've been meaning to read.

2. I have a 'when brain gone' list to make sure I can still be productive on days where anything intellectual is not going to happen.

3. I enjoy the 'incubate' table, where I put things I know I'll do one day. There's a perfect time for things like writing books or starting a Master's course, but they might need to mature for a while.

4. The 'someday/maybe' table is for things that would be good to do at some point, but aren't certainties. So for me, this includes dreams like attending a midwifery conference in the USA, visiting my partner's family in Florida, etc.

5. I try to stay really relaxed about how much I get done on any one day. This system means as long as you keep an eye on your calendar and your to-do list, everything eventually gets done. Think flexibility – we do yoga to stay loose and not get hurt, we have an editable to-do list for the same reason.

Big picture time management tools

Now you have a way of recording and planning your tasks, there are some time management tools you may find helpful in giving you an overview of how your midwifery training is going.

1. Gantt charts are great for when you want to visualize all your deadlines and how things cross over and interact. I make mine via Monday.com; I don't need to make many of them so their free trial works out well.

2. You can use Trello for visually mapping things out; see Chapters Seven and Eight for examples.

3. Use email scheduler tools. These are useful because you can deal with emails from tutors, etc., as soon as they come into your inbox, without being that annoying person who emails back straight away. You can also set yourself reminders. I use Boomerang which is on Gmail but there are others. I believe Deskrun is free.

4. Organize your office space. There are loads of good guides around: Marie Kondo is great, as is the guide in *Getting Things Done* (Allen 2015: part 2). If someone had tried to get me to organize myself when I was a student midwife I probably would have said some-thing like 'I'm sure that works for some people', i.e. I would have been passive-aggressive about how that was a bad use of time. But this meant by the end of my degree I had lots of big box files which had random badly folded bits of paper in them, and when I needed to find certain lecture notes, handouts or other important papers like student loan documents, I'd have to dig through everything I owned and get hot and anxious about where things were. These days I like to spend a few hours with my filing cabinet with a podcast on in the background. If you spend some time setting up a system, and every so often do some maintenance on it, you'll save so much time, but more importantly, you'll be more enthusiastic about any given task you need to start.

    When you process your in list (or just when you feel like it) you may want to use the following questions. If it feels too heavy, maybe not. But they can be helpful in the right moment.

Gantt chart from Monday.com

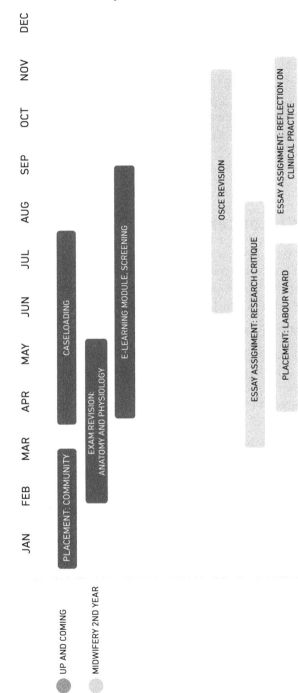

MIDWIFERY 2023

UP AND COMING

MIDWIFERY 2ND YEAR

JAN FEB MAR APR MAY JUN JUL AUG SEP OCT NOV DEC

PLACEMENT: COMMUNITY

CASELOADING

EXAM REVISION: ANATOMY AND PHYSIOLOGY

E-LEARNING MODULE, SCREENING

OSCE REVISION

ESSAY ASSIGNMENT: RESEARCH CRITIQUE

PLACEMENT: LABOUR WARD

ESSAY ASSIGNMENT: REFLECTION ON CLINICAL PRACTICE

Box 1.4: Exciting career questions

What are my longer-term goals for my career?

What projects (assignments, personal reading) should I have in place to make sure I'm pursuing these?

What other significant opportunities or events are happening in my midwifery degree/in midwifery as a whole that could offer me options?

What projects should I set up to help me take advantage of these?

Help with concentration

We all have days when we feel completely useless. I get so frustrated with myself and it is incredibly normal to feel like this. Everything takes longer than it should and my standard reply when my partner asks how my day is going is 'I'm getting very little done'.

Here are some ideas to help:

1. Take one small task and finish it. Just a small amount of forward motion can get you back into a positive mindset. To do this, take a single piece of paper and write your task on it. Have this and your materials for it out only. Concentrate on just one thing at a time.

2. Sleep is essential. A friend of mine who is a successful lawyer went to Cambridge University, where she had to write an essay each week. After doing all her research she would go to bed and always wake up halfway through the night with her essay strategy solved. I've tried this and I'm not the kind of person who wakes up with a perfect essay in my head, but sleep does mean I'm rested, I have a fresh perspective and quite a lot of the time I've made connections between ideas that will be useful for the assignment.

3. If you're confused about your task and your brain keeps telling you to go and do something else, you have a couple of options. The first is to continue for at least an hour while keeping a piece of paper next to you to write down any other tasks that pop into

your head. Or you can stop and do a review of your tasks and see if you would indeed be better off spending time on something else. Do as much planning as you need to get planning off your mind.

4. Set an alarm for an hour. During that hour you are only allowed to work on the task you've set yourself or look out of the window. No Twitter, Facebook, etc.

5. The Pomodoro technique suggests working for 25 minutes, with a 5-minute break. Do this for 30 minutes then give yourself half an hour off. I find this works sometimes but it's horribly prescriptive other times. Remember as a profession we're unhealthy with breaks, so catch yourself before you burn out.

For emergencies – if midwifery and life has become unmanageable

- Midwives I have interviewed about postgraduate work often talked to me about needing extensions; is this a time you need one?

- If life has just gone a bit nuts and you need a way through in the short term, write down what you need to get done – the non-negotiables. This is your calendar list for the next day. Preferably, limit yourself to three tasks, or six at the very most.

- Know that sometimes we get through but we have no idea how we managed it. I think it's normal to hit at least one of these times during midwifery training.

Jess' to-do list

One of my friends is Jess Wood, a second-year on a four-year Master's course and has two little ones under the age of five. I thought she'd be a good example to draw from and I've processed her in list as if it's my own.

Box 1.5: Jess' in list

study BFI breastfeeding complexities

caseloading appointments and births

Midwifery society

systematic physical examination of the newborn (SPEN) e-learning

buy Paeds stethoscope for NIPE/SPEN

leadership portfolio

leadership learning set meetings
self-directed study on The Eye, Sensory

Disabilities, Evidence-based practice
read guidelines on diabetes, cardiac disease, multiple pregnancy,
anaemia & haemoglobinopathies, social determinants of health

read MBRRACE reports

make study guides for A + P of: anaemia, cardiac disorders, diabetes,
multiple pregnancy

critique 3 studies for strengths/weaknesses for EBP

arrange 2nd formative review with practice assessor

prepare for placement in 2 weeks

book Beyond Bea study day

book SANDS webinar

EBP essay 2000 words

study for NIPE/SPEN OSCE

study for complex care & infant feeding exam

write Gibbs reflections on placement

get MORA competencies signed off
online and face-to-face lectures

rewrite first year notes

get women's feedback in MORA

running as part of our Nursing/Midwifery fundraiser

2nd COVID vaccine

choose a research topic

keep up to date with maternity current events

look into prerequisites for midwife jobs abroad

arrange childcare around my eldest

starting school in September

find a new nursery for the younger one

keep the Husband sane

learn Arabic

eat well

exercise

Vitamins

car MOT

renew passports

Cat food

Quilt

anniversary

Reflect on (emotional well-being);

Doctor interaction on 14th, ask cohort

Supervisor – am I being sensitive or just hard? Ask Hina, she's been there ...

Run marathon

DIY re-do bathroom and lounge

Catalogue phone images

Table 1.3: Jess' processed to-do list

Type of Task	Begin with ...	Defer until ...
Urgent		
Put new lecture timetable into calendar		
Book 2nd Covid vaccine		
Wash uniforms		

Jobs to Do When Tired		
Bulk buy cat food	Price compare	Get paid on Friday

Family Jobs		
Childcare	Research nursery and childminder around school	
Date night	Add to calendar	
Renew passports	Research how we do this online	

Anniversary		...
1st Sept	Choose film + restaurant	New restaurant guide published

Health Jobs		...
Running	Calendar for running	Running shoes arrive
Supplements	Research – ?fish oil	Finished antibiotics

Life Admin		
Car MOT	Call garage	8am Saturday

Hobbies/Fun		
Quilting	Research what to buy	
Learn Arabic	Find app	

Assignments		
Systematic physical examination of the newborn (SPEN) e-learning	Find log ins; try first quiz to see how much study is needed; choose top 20% of topics to start flashcards for NIPE/SPEN	Internet upgrade complete

Type of Task	Begin with ...	Defer until ...
Leadership portfolio	List top 20% of what needs to be in there; collect certificates from emails	
Evidence-Based Learning	Choose 3 studies for critique strengths/weaknesses for EBP Split 2000 words into categories	
Gibbs reflection	Choose skill	
Research topic for dissertation	Choose topic	Two weeks into placement when topic has come up ... (20th Sept? ...)
Reading and mind map ideas	Think on train	Journey to Birmingham conf.

Exams		
Physiology of eye	Find notes; top 20% onto revision cards	
make study guides for A + P for: anaemia, cardiac disorders, diabetes, multiple pregnancy	Review notes, review textbook chapter, top 20% onto flashcards	Month before exam (2nd Oct)
study BFI breastfeeding complexities	Mindmap areas I need to expand knowledge on; use BFI curriculum checklist, top 20% onto flashcards	Month before exam (2nd Oct)

Degree (miscellaneous jobs)		
Leadership learning set meetings	Email personal tutor	
Evidence-based practice learning	Find recent book and schedule reading time	
Sensory disabilities	Find 1x personal blog, 1x outside agency resource and 1x research paper on subject	After Birmingham conf.
Read MBRRACE reports	Find which ones from NPEU website	
Book Beyond Bea and SANDS study day	Look at dates	Get paid
Keep up to date with maternity current events	Spend an hour subscribing to blogs	

Type of Task	Begin with ...	Defer until ...
Degree (admin jobs)		
Arrange 2nd formative review with practice assessor	Email possible dates to assessor	

Caseloading		
Find clients to follow through	Put course dates in diary, fit appointments around, decide on-call hours	

Career Advancement		
Look into prerequisites for midwife jobs abroad	Research agencies	Exam date given for Sept

Placement		
Read guidelines on diabetes, cardiac disease, multiple pregnancy, anaemia & haemoglobinopathies, social determinants of health	Download guidelines on placement and email to self; make notes on top 20% of content	Can request some time on placement when workload is appropriate
Midwifery Ongoing Record of Achievement (MORA) proficiencies signed off	Go through MORA, bookmark for different areas and decide on the easiest to focus on first; (women feedback?)	

Things to Buy		
Paediatric stethoscope	Price compare	
Budgeting Jobs		
Tesco – delivery subscription	Price compare supermarket deliveries	

Emotional Well-being		
Midwifery society	Look up meet dates on FB, sign up	Jane confirms she's coming
Supervisor – am I being sensitive or just hard?	Ask Hina, she's been there ...	The moment feels right

Someday/Maybe		
Midwifery in India		

Type of Task	Begin with ...	Defer until ...
Incubate		
DIY re-do bathroom and lounge		
Print and catalogue photos from phone		

To conclude

There's a contradiction in this chapter, as in the Introduction I said that you should only implement what feels right to you and then I followed up with a lot of precise strategies to try. The to-do list method and all the other tools in this chapter are useful, and I've been able to get things done faster or with less difficulty using them, but these days I'm more slack about following every step and I just do what works. You are your own person, use them as a prompt rather than a prescription.

Essays

Introduction

A lot of students find essays difficult because you have to concentrate on two things: you need to be involved with the details while still knowing how the piece is going as a whole. It's hard to keep both of these in mind while you're also understanding new material and working out how to write academically. In this chapter, we'll think about why essays exist and why they can be daunting, and some strategies to help. We'll move on to getting clear on what your assignment question is asking you to do, and finding new useful ideas from resources on your reading list and further afield. Then we'll think about how to ensure you are including critical analysis, how to structure an essay and make an essay plan, and how to write it up.

Why essays exist

At the beginning of the Enlightenment, the writer Montaigne started to publish ideas under the title 'essays'. The word 'essay' translates in French as 'to try or attempt'. This was a new concept because before this the focus of scholarly writing was on teaching or offering proof, as opposed to using the form itself as a way of logically exploring a topic. There were many people writing about academic ideas before Montaigne came along; he was drawing from Plutarch, who in turn had learnt from the logic of early Islamic scholars. But Montaigne does seem to have popularized the modern essay as a form. Essay writing caught on in Europe, and travelled through the sciences, impacting Shakespeare and many other notable thinkers, until they became part of the way students were tested on their learning (Williams 2020).

Essays aren't actually about showing off your knowledge and cramming in references so you get a good grade. They're about tackling difficult questions and trying to come up with some useful conclusions. They're a way of thinking through your arguments, and the clearer you can make things for your reader, the clearer the ideas will become to yourself. In midwifery, where clients rely on us to give them balanced information so they can make critically important decisions, being able to assess the research and communicate your point of view is important.

Essay writing is also an art form. You need to summon a piece of work into existence using a series of judgement calls around what to include and at what level of detail. Most study guides won't lead with this point. I think they're concerned that you'll forget the evidence if they talk about creativity. But though we should aim to be as objective as possible when writing academically, all knowledge is contestable and there is no certainty. This means what you're attempting with an essay assignment is creativity, with all the psychological challenges that comes with that. I hope knowing all this will help you see the beauty of putting together information in this way.

An overview

A sensible path through essay writing looks something like this:

Assess Question > Read Material > Choose Points > Critique Material > Structure Outline > Write

But in reality, writing an essay is an iterative and fluid process. The different stages will spill into each other as you consider things more deeply or go back and change your mind. It looks a bit more like this, but with more arrows:

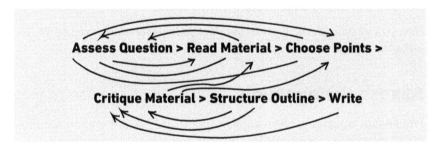

It can feel like Spaghetti Junction. There is no perfect way of doing things. I questioned every single sentence I wrote in this chapter; every instruction is up for debate. And a piece of writing is never finished, you just decide to cut it off and move on.

Your process

As I said earlier, I'd argue that essay writing is a creative task. You start with a blank page, and though you need to write factually, the material you choose to discuss and critique will create a unique piece of work. This is possibly why many people don't go near their essays until late on, it's their brain telling them not to engage with uncertainty (uncertain homo erectus got eaten). You'll need to create some mental space and you might well benefit from a process of some kind. A process is a set of actions you do to achieve something complex.

Creative processes tend to be personal to us and come with a particular environment and you will probably have an idea of what your process is from previous academic or creative work. For instance, it might be that to get started you have to choose your literature and then take it for a walk, stopping in cafes to read for periods of time, thinking and writing between stops. I know one student who is best off at her desk but needs to be using a fidget toy because she can't concentrate without being physically engaged. And I like to get my books at the library and then go home because my most productive place for reading and notetaking is lying on my floor on this roll out mattress thing my sister bought me.

You need to hit the place where you're concentrating, which might come with some emotions like doubt or confusion because you're working with new material, but you should also be interested, and you shouldn't be panicked. Settling into a task takes time, so your process should take the edge off while you're beginning to engage. Part of my process includes setting up a Google document. This is where I'll make voice notes. I'll make a shortcut for it on the homepage of my phone, because ideas often pop up while I'm doing something else and the aim is to capture them fast before I forget. I might also start a mind map and/or a page of handwritten ideas.

Now you've considered how to support your psychology, we can move on to the assignment question.

Assess the question

I find essay questions often appear simple at first, but the more I think about them, the more complex they get. For instance, let's take a question like:

Box 2.1: Sample essay question

Describe the physiological changes that take place during the process of establishing breastfeeding. Discuss the role of the midwife when providing care to clients during the puerperium in relation to breastfeeding.

When getting to the heart of what the question means, there will be specific words to identify. Have a look at the table below what a few possible academic terms are prompting you to do (check your university library online resources; it's likely they will have a comprehensive version of this table which is freely available to you.)

Table 2.1: Definitions of instruction words for essay writing*

Analyse	Break down into component parts. Examine critically or closely.
Comment on/criticize/ evaluate/ critically evaluate/assess	Judge the value of something. But first, analyse, describe and explain. Then go through the arguments for and against, laying out the arguments neutrally until the section where you make your judgement clear. Judgements should be backed by reasons and evidence.
Compare/contrast/ distinguish/ differentiate/relate	All these require that you discuss how things are related to each other. Compare suggests you concentrate on similarities, which may lead to a stated preference, the justification of which should be made clear. These words suggest that two situations or ideas can be compared in a number of different ways, or from a variety of viewpoints. Contrast suggests you concentrate on differences.
Define	Write down the precise meaning of a word or phrase. Sometimes several co-existing definitions may be used and, possibly, evaluated.

From this we can pick out:

- Describe = give a detailed account of.
- Discuss = consider; decide what the main issues are.

So far so good. But when you consider further, what exactly is your tutor looking for? Antenatal education provision? Psychology? Physiology, clearly, but how much detail? Sociology? How much word count should you allocate to each topic? The role of a midwife is a key concept. Breastfeeding is *the* key topic. How do you get all of this in?

If you get concerned about not knowing exactly what your tutor is asking for, you're bang on target. The complexity is about getting you to think deeply. At this stage, you'll come up with lots of ways of answering, and then you can choose which of your best thoughts when you put your outline together.

1. One way of tackling an essay question is to try to write it out in your own words. They're dense questions, so you'll probably go into quite a bit of detail. It's a good idea to include keywords that have been covered in lectures.

   For instance if we take our example question again:

*(Adapted from University of Bath 2020)

Box 2.2: An essay question unpacked

Describe the physiological changes that take place during the process of establishing breastfeeding. Discuss the role of the midwife when providing care to clients during the puerperium in relation to breastfeeding.

Overall this means: describe the establishment of breastfeeding/chestfeeding, specifically around the way the body changes. And discuss the role of the midwife in relation to breastfeeding/chestfeeding over the first 6–8 weeks of the postnatal period.

Relevant concepts include the changes the body makes. For instance lactogenesis, alveoli cells, oestrogen, progesterone and prolactin, oxytocin and the letdown reflex, and so on.

Midwives have to know about physiological changes to provide good care that covers the minds and bodies of clients, babies, families and the wider community.

This is because excellent evidence-based information comes from what we know about physiology. Information about this needs to be delivered to women and birthing people in a way they can understand. This helps support informed decisions and contributes to holistic care.

Holistic means 'intimately connected and can only be referred to in terms of the whole'. Aspects of care to do with psychology and sociology are linked and back each other up in complex ways. But overall this question is asking if I can describe the physiological changes. The focus needs to be on the physical side of things.

The second part of the question relates to the postnatal period up to 8 weeks (the puerperium). Most midwives hand care to health visitors around 10 days, so there's possibly an organization of care/care provision angle to discuss.

The question might also be asking about whether midwives giving care further into the postnatal period could help with breastfeeding rates, something we have challenges with in the UK. Certainly, the role of the midwife does include the promotion of public health which breastfeeding/chestfeeding is part of. But the first part of the question is all about the establishment of breastfeeding/chestfeeding so perhaps this question is about how excellent early care can support physiology and improve rates that way.

2. Once I've unpacked the question in this manner, I might then have a look through any example essays I've been given (there will usually be at least one provided to help you). I'll add to my notes, thinking about what they've done well and what to avoid.

3. Then I'll have a good look at the mark scheme, taking note of any specifications. Mark schemes can be unspecific, but there might be hints like 'judgement' and 'synthesize' which you can think about.

4. Once I've done all this, I like to progress my thinking a little further. Writing out statements that challenge aspects of the assignment title or seeing the problem from alternative angles can be useful. Sometimes I'll even choose keywords from the question and use an online antonym dictionary (antonym meaning a word opposite in meaning) to prompt ideas. For instance, some ideas that are in opposition to the question are:

    a. What are the psychological, rather than physiological, changes which take place during early breastfeeding/chestfeeding?
    b. What would be poor practice around midwifery care and breastfeeding/chestfeeding in the 6–8 weeks after birth?
    c. Is it equally important to offer care to those not breastfeeding/chestfeeding? How would a midwife offer care that supports the physiology of those choosing to formula feed?
    d. Are there important bits of this process that happen during the antenatal period?
    e. What are the commonly held truths about supporting breast-feeding/chestfeeding as a midwife that are uncontested? Can I pull these ideas apart? What's wrong with them?

5. Once I've unpacked the task I write out what I feel are the key parts. I might put them on an A4 piece of paper and stick it above my desk to help myself stay on track.

6. If you have feedback from your last essay and you think you've identified a strength or weakness to keep in mind, stick this up as well.

By this stage I will have a group of diverse first thoughts; this might mean a handwritten sheet of A4, a word document full of notes, and/or a mind map. Now you are familiar with the territory and have a starting point, you'll need to expand your knowledge.

> *Breastfeeding/chestfeeding physiology*
> *– body changes and anatomy*
>
> *Holistic care*
>
> *midwife's handover to health visitor (briefly)*
>
> *Public health and breastfeeding (briefly)*
>
> *Don't get stuck on just one topic!*

Finding and reading material

Remember the Spaghetti Junction image from the beginning of this chapter that showed how writing an essay involves the different tasks overlapping and looping back on each other? The finding and reading materials stage is a good example of this. You might start by getting a general overview from a few books on the reading list, go on to find more detailed or up-to-date sources using your library catalogue, read some recent research and then find gaps in your knowledge where you'll need to look at the basic texts from the reading list again, then go back and search for more using a different angle ... it's all up to you and your method will depend on your preferences, the essay task and how the project goes.

Reading lists

Reading lists are a guide for you to follow through the wide range of possible reading you could do. Some students report feeling frustrated at the idea of a reading list because they can't do their own thing. This is understandable, and actually quite a good instinct as you need to do some literature searching in order to access higher marks. But considering that the tutors who set the essay are usually the same people who wrote the reading list, it's a good idea to at least start there.

> I spend my entire assignment scouring for sources and when finished go back and realize I could have saved a lot of time if I'd started with the reading list! But I also find it's not really possible to stick only to their lists and achieve the best marks.
>
> **Amy Eloise Walsh**

If you're struggling because what you're reading is new to you and you're confused, you may want to start with a blog or article designed to summarize or introduce you to the subject. Another issue that can crop up is that reading lists can be long and intimidating. If you've got a huge list and you know you won't get through all of it, you may want to ask your tutors which book they'd start with if they were just getting to know the topic. You can also use 80/20: what are the top 20 per cent of books or resources that look most likely to be helpful? You can then look at the top 20 per cent of the content of each book.

Finally, the SQR3 technique is good for speed reading. This stands for S – survey; Q – form questions; R – read; R – recite; R – review. The idea is you flick through a book to get your bearings, and while you do this you start to form questions about the content. Then you read through in detail and answer your questions, if you can. The finals Rs, recite and review, are about repeating what you've learned to get it fixed in your mind. All of this should help you retain much more information. Check out a Khan Academy post on SQR3 for further details (Khan Academy 2018).

Searching for sources on your own

When choosing material to read, you'll need a few different techniques. Some of them are common sense; for instance, you might know of a book chapter on the subject from other reading you've been doing, or someone in practice might have mentioned something important. But your mind map or notes from your assessment of the question will also have generated topics, ideas and keywords. You can use these to search.

You are likely to have had a session on how to use your library's resources and now would be the time to put these skills into practice. This stage might involve searching widely using Google, then more specifically using your library catalogue, or even more niche would be searching a midwifery journal.

When searching and using keywords, think about the following:

- Is this keyword about the question?
- Is it biased?
- How is knowledge changing?
- What are the different points of view?
- What is your point of view and can you defend it?
- Is it likely that things will change in the future?

These are complex questions and you won't be able to answer them in detail, they're just to stimulate your thinking.

There's a more formal way of searching for materials, known as a literature search. This involves keywords and searching through reference lists of particular sources, and keeping records of what you searched for, and you'll get onto this later in your degree. There's no end to how exacting you can be about searching but for most undergraduate assignments you just need to show engagement with relevant sources. Many academic writers reflecting on their degree course will say you should aim for about one peer-reviewed reference for every 200 words you write (Squirrell 2020). So for a 2,000-word essay, a couple of books, 5–10 articles (some that you read in-depth and some that you skim), a couple of bits of 'grey literature' in the form of government reports, and a piece of material like a news article would be a good shout.

Have a look at the table for the possible types of material you could find. I wish I could be more specific and include names of clinical bodies and so on but it will differ depending on where you are in the world.

Table 2.2: Resources to find evidence for essays

Lectures and seminars	Charity guides	Professional reflections
Conversations with tutors and others	Legislation	Grand rounds
Books	Governing body publications	Academic or clinical models and theories
Theses	Healthcare Professional Codes	Journal articles
Conferences	The World Health Organization	Books and textbooks
Agency publications	Social media	Newspapers
Hospital guidelines	The Cochrane Library	Government papers
The Cochrane Library	Podcasts	National guidelines
National and international statistics	Professional YouTube channels or other videos	Database searches
Client perspectives and stories	Ebooks	Clinical guidelines

Further reading ideas

- Getting an up-to-date copy of a comprehensive midwifery text-book (in the UK that would mean Mayes or Myles) and finding a relevant chapter is a good place to start, particularly if an essay is on physiology or a practical clinical skill – lots of universities now give you e-copies of these for free.
- If you're in the library and you find one good book, have a look at the shelf and see what else is there.

- Reviewing your notes on lectures will help you cover your bases.

- You can look at the example essay or talk to your tutor to understand the scope of what you're being asked to do, but I'd try and go above and beyond as well.

- Many will hate this suggestion but Wikipedia can be a good place to get an idea of where you're headed. Just check the sources and reference those rather than referencing Wikipedia itself.

- You should also choose some of the texts on the reading list you've been given and read them using the SQR3 method, or another method that helps you read quickly and easily.

- Mixing things up with videos can be great as just reading can get very tiring. Remember on YouTube you can often click the three dots below the video and get a transcript which you can then search through or quote from more easily (and find out the keyboard shortcut to search through a page of text for a particular word: Google 'search keyboard shortcut' and the name of your device, it takes seconds to work out how to do it and it will save you so much time).

- Going for a walk and listening to a podcast can be a restorative way of researching which gives you the energy to write.

- You will often get tipped off about good pieces of research by reading journal articles and looking at their reference lists, though be aware that following things back can be an unending rabbit hole.

- As you begin to crack the spine of this essay, you'll likely feel some opinions coming together. There's a whole other stage where you can critique material in detail, so don't worry about coming to firm conclusions yet. But ideally, you should be following your curiosity.

This brings us to the end of this stage and your initial dive into the reading. After you've considered the different types of materials you could look at, you should feel like you could have a go at writing the essay, but also you'll have lots more questions. However, many students, tutors and librarians will tell you this stage often comes to an end simply because of time pressure, which is fine. Essentially, it's a judgement call between feeling like you know enough and being aware of your deadline (Clarke 2020).

Note taking

As you work through your books and other resources, you'll need to keep notes on any good bits of critique or cool ideas you have. Make consistent notes linked to the reference, i.e. if you think you're going to quote directly, make sure you have the page number and author's name. You can set up Zotero or Mendeley or another referencing management tool (you can Google how to do this), which will make you a reference list for your essay.

I like to take notes with a word document open, using my phone and voice transcription software. I also use voice search to find definitions or further clarification on things I'm not sure about and I might also write certain ideas on a mind map or handwrite notes onto an A4 pad. The point is to keep a record while not getting pulled out of what you're reading.

Choose points

In terms of choosing how many points to make in your essay, you'll first need to consider word count.

For a 2,000-word essay, the following is about right.

Box 2.3: Essay word count

10%/200 words for introduction
80%/1,600 words for main body
10%/200 words for conclusion

You will likely need between one and three paragraphs to explain each point and the evidence backing it up. This means for a 2,000-word essay, you'll need perhaps 200 words to cover an introduction, which leaves 200–400 words per point. This equals around five key points you can make in the main body of your essay. A point might be an argument, a description or a critique of the evidence. You don't have to commit to these points entirely but I'd narrow it down if you can. There will always be a lot more you could say in your essay, so the points you settle on come down to a judgement call. You just need to choose some areas to concentrate on so you know what to read and critique in more detail.

At this point, you'll probably have a lot of unprocessed notes in the form of mind maps, word documents or, if you're anything like me, misspelt and slightly hard to decipher ideas recorded using voice to text software. Hopefully, they will all have references (I tend to write the book or resource title into my notes page **bold and underlined** so I can see the reference for each idea). You can now go through and circle a few key points that you know should be in your essay. Look at your mark scheme and your original assessment of the question; what deserves the most attention? You should also think about what warrants further reading and critique. Write these points on a new piece of paper or type them into a word document.

Skills for midwifery practice:

involution considered more likely with BF

temp rises physiologically with BF women 3rd day pn

glandular tissue, ductal network, alveoli, lactocytes, myoepithelial cells, oxytocin, muscle contraction – milk through ducts on demand, not stored

colostrum from 16th week, loss of placental hormones, mainly progest. + oxytocin = milk comes in

early priming through oxytocin promoting skin to skin etc. important for long-term supply

Midwifery Skills at a Glance:

feeding cues

reduced chance of cancer, pnd, osteoporosis

nipples no damage, oxytocin signs like afterpains breastcrawl

express first to encourage

responsive feeding

Roar Behind silence:

Partners attending bf class = greater uptake

Amy Brown Paper lessons BF:

normal rather than best

family member support

TV ads?

NHS Start for Life:

emphasis on colic? not normality?

alcohol not encouraged, conflicts evidence A.Brown as not much goes through? – but SIDS

bonding/lovely> expectations? calories – body image, negative

glandular tissue, ductal network alveoli, lactocytes, myoepithelial cells, oxytocin, muscle contraction – milk through ducts on demand, not stored

loss of placental hormones, mainly progest. + oxytocin = milk comes in

early priming through oxytocin promoting skin to skin etc. important for long-term supply

reduced chance of cancer, pnd, osteoporosis (skills mw practice)

nipples no damage, breastcrawl, responsive feeding (skills glance)

partners attending bf class = greater uptake (RBS)

bonding, lovely, body image, contrast with real experience (NHS best start, Brown paper)

(I've tidied this example up a bit, but you get the picture).

Critique material

You should now have a few journal articles that you want to read more closely and appraise. For me, this bit is fun and exciting but also really hard. There are certain guidelines you can use for research appraisal but it's essentially something you'll have to work on and develop throughout your career. It can feel like you're under pressure because the more critical evaluation you can get into your essay, the higher the marks available. The thing to remember is that no one is expecting you to singlehandedly find a gaping hole in methodologically conducted studies published by the top global multidisciplinary research units or anything even similar to this. I think I had some grandiose ideas about this kind of thing when I was an undergrad, but, y'know, leave something in case you want to do a PhD.

What might be a more achievable aim for this stage is to understand the paper or other source as well as you possibly can. Would you be able to explain the research and findings to a layperson, say your partner or mum? Then as your understanding grows and you gain some knowledge around your chosen topic and appreciation for the choices the researchers or author has made, you'll be able to see some of the issues with the material. You may then find yourself giving some suggestions around how you might fix those issues.

For instance, say you've got three sources you want to read in depth as part of the preparation for a 2,000-word essay. It will also be important to check what other experts in the field are saying to see if they are in agreement with you.

Some of the questions you can ask yourself are:

- Are any assumptions being made in this text?
- Assumptions might include:

  _____ is important.

  _____ is possible.

  _____ might influence _____.

  _____ is a positive thing.

  _____ is a negative thing.

- Do these assumptions seem reasonable in this context? Why or why not?
- Do any claims seem too certain?
- Are there suitable examples?

- Are there claims which are based on authority for support? What kind of authority is it? Does this seem reasonable?
- Are there claims which are based on evidence for support? What kind of evidence is it? Does this seem reasonable?
- What is missing from the text?
- How could the text be not like this/different?
- Are any groups being excluded or marginalized in the text or in the implications of the claims?
- What would the implications be if we were to take the claims seriously? i.e. what would happen next?
- What else? (Can you think of further critical questions? Do you have a favourite question?)

(University College London (UCL) 2018)

Pick a few questions that spark your interest or seem to go somewhere. You could also use a basic guide to interpreting research – your university should have recommended one and might have a publication that's specific to midwifery in mind. You can also see Chapter Six, 'Engaging with Research', in this book for more information.

For your first few essays or assignments, most of what you write will be demonstrating you know the topic and have understood what you have been reading, with only a little critique of sources you've read. As you progress through your course, the weight will shift towards including more research appraisal. While this might

Box 2.4: How to keep notes while doing research appraisal

Having photocopied chapters of books or printed out research papers from journals can be useful if you like to annotate and highlight key areas. But students report it's easy to turn off when doing this. It feels like you're doing something active but if you're highlighting big chunks of text and not reflecting much, be suspicious (Young 2020). As with your initial reading, put points you're considering covering in your essay into your notes, with the reference included so you know where the idea came from.

be too prescriptive for some, I know of one academic who suggests by the third year of a degree, criticism and appraisal should make up about one-quarter of your essay content (Yonis 2018).

As you think further about the source in front of you, you'll begin to see that you need to go for depth, not breadth. The problem with this is you're new to the field. You haven't got time to become an expert so while you're reading you'll have to make some educated guesses about what's going on. It's a vulnerable process because, honestly, you might well get some things wrong. You're a small fish in an extremely big sea. But in my experience, the one thing tutors find depressing is a student who doesn't want to commit to what they *actually* think. You might be a little fish, but they'll like it if you're a brave one.

All of this thinking in the critique stage might require a few different sessions and you might need to give yourself time and space. Your process might well come into play here. One of my researcher friends keeps a notebook by the side of her bed as she has interesting ideas in the middle of the night. Researcher and independent midwife Dr Sara Wickham says she does this as well (Wickham 2015: 922). The aim is to add worthy ideas to your word document, written notes or mind map.

Structure outline

You should now have a huge field of ideas or possible points to make in the form of your word document, mind map or written notes, with an easy way of referencing where they're from. I would then think about where they might fit into your essay.

A good outline will mean a good structure, with one point leading to the next idea. There should be a clear connection between each point, and your writing should be building towards something in a 'tight chain of reasoning' (McCool 2009: 2). As discussed, for a 2,000-word essay, you'll need about five main points. You'll now need to work out what order to put them in.

I get to my structure by printing out my notes and cutting out the points I've chosen to focus on, as well as a lot of the supporting evidence and other ideas I think will be important to include. I then move the points and other ideas around on my floor until I'm happy with the order.

I will also get rid of some ideas that don't fit into the assignment well – for instance, if I have a point that's more of a description and the essay is asking me to analyse, I might discard it. Melissa Newman, a midwife who is undertaking her doctorate right now, refers to the 'golden thread' which holds an essay together, meaning there is one single concept that builds the narrative. However, there can be different ways to structure your outline – for instance, grouped by theme, or say you're looking at how practice has changed over time, it might make sense to do things chronologically.

For me, there's something about the tactile nature of this kind of cutting-out project, and almost being inside the structure, that helps me to find an outline. I then Blu Tack my points in order on my wall or take a picture of the order with my phone. For planning bigger projects like this book I now Blu Tack the points to boards that I buy off eBay. This technique might be helpful if you're planning a bigger piece of writing like a dissertation.

My floor technique might be a little over-engineered for you, but there are lots of other ways of building an outline. You can, of course, do it on a computer and move the points around a word document. I know some students who use a big roll of parcel paper with different

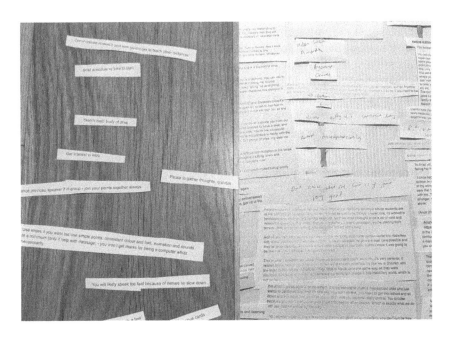

coloured pens. When I ask how they come to a conclusion about the order of their points the answer is 'it just feels like it should go there'. I think the idea is they write points out with lots of space around them so they can fill in and order their outline as they work through their ideas.

My friend Kristie actually starts writing before this point and doesn't bother about an outline. She moves the sections of her essay around once she's written them to find a good flow. And having talked with Oxbridge students who have to churn out an essay each week, it seems they don't worry too much about amassing lots of points before choosing what goes in. They seem to do some reading, pick a few ideas, get a basic order down and run with it (Williams 2020). If any of these ideas work for you, great. But most of us doing an undergraduate midwifery degree will need to spend time thinking about an outline and will use a workflow to get to it.

If some ideas occur to you that will help you write a crisp, short introduction, then add them to the top of your outline. You should also be coming to some decisions about your conclusion because you've done so much reading and considering. But don't be concerned if you aren't at this stage yet, you can always write these in after writing the rest of your essay.

If you're allowed, send a small section of your essay draft to your tutor. A standard allowance is 500 words, but check with your university. It may be helpful to choose the weakest area, so they can offer constructive feedback. I hear many universities subscribe to an ethical feedback website/service called 'Studiosity', so do check. In addition, academic skills advisers, usually found via university libraries, are also good at checking through essay plans. If there are any major problems with your essay, it's best to hear them early. Very few students will do this and I wish I had more.

Remember our essay question:

> 'Describe the physiological changes that take place during the process of establishing breastfeeding. Discuss the role of the midwife when providing care to clients during the puerperium in relation to breastfeeding.

Here is an example essay plan.

Essay Plan

Physiological changes over initiation of bf

glandular tissue, ductal network, alveoli, lactocytes, myoepithelial cells, oxytocin, muscle contraction – milk through ducts on demand, not stored, loss of placental hormones, mainly progesterone + oxytocin = milk comes in

(critique what we know, oligosaccharides fed by bf<microbiome>but we don't know much yet, e.g. mycobiome – oligosaccharides (Borewicz)

challenge cs/instrumental (Banks)

Physiological changes over first 6–8 weeks

expectations; 6 weeks to get working well (Minchin); support team, positioning (Banks)

Block feeding, 8 weeks, pain from arched palate, small mouth, infection tongue tie if continues by this point? Misinformation and lack of knowledge re thrush (glycogen in tissues, microbiome) (BF network)

Midwife's role supporting physiology mentioned above

early priming through oxytocin promoting skin to skin etc. important for long-term supply, nipples no damage, breastcrawl, responsive feeding (skills glance)

Partners attending bf class = greater uptake (RBS)

confidence building after difficult birth (Mercer, Hendricks)

Public health

reduced chance of cancer, pnd, osteoporosis (skills mw practice)

bonding, lovely, body image, contrast with real experience (NHS best start, Brown paper)

educating friends and family, empowerment, groups (Dudzinska)

What we don't know/do well

LGBTQ + particularly transgender and non-binary clients and support – producing milk (Reisman, Goldstein)

peer support; 'caught not taught' (Mayo)

flexible working hours, but sex discrimination continues – health and safety law, discrimination law (mat action, Gettas)

Write

Now you've done your preparation, you can write up. In the writing stage, you get to bring your own voice to the project.

What you're aiming for is a bit like a completed jigsaw. The whole thing together is uniform, of the same tone and makes a smooth picture, but you can also see each individual piece, by which I mean the evidence you're citing. You can achieve this by describing the research and arguments you've read using phrases like 'this shows ...', 'the work criticizes ...', 'this study concludes ...' and so on, and also by keeping everything objective. Objective means factual, so pretend you're reading your essay to a very critical friend or family member who isn't interested in your feelings or point of view. They just want the evidence, as far as can be achieved (you can also imagine you're reading to Spock).

You can also reference concepts, theories and models.

Box 2.5: Concepts, theories and models

A quick note on this. A concept is a 'general idea or notion'; a theory is 'abstract knowledge or principles, as opposed to practical experience or activity' (Scanlan et al. 2013: 33); and a model is 'an abstract representation upon which a discipline is based' (Bryar and Sinclair 2011: 28).

Concepts are pretty straightforward, they're just ideas, usually abstract ones like 'pain is often a feature of childbirth'. But the definition of a theory is more complex. It's different from a fact because it's contestable, but it has been researched thoroughly. Theories can be more or less accepted but are still evidence-based ways of thinking about things. For instance Bryar and Sinclair cite Grantly Dick-Read as documenting the fear/tension cycle that can cause complications in childbirth (2011: 28).

A model is even more complicated, as it's a removed way of looking at things that might involve different frameworks, bits of information and insights being put together in an organized fashion. They can be useful in healthcare as they give us a way of understanding how we give care and the system supporting it; for instance, midwives often work within the 'partnership model' of care which is to do with being women/client-centred. Models can be described using language, or through pictures or diagrams (Bryar and Sinclair 2011: 29, 304).

You can use concepts, theories and models in your essays because they are ways of examining complex ideas. There are whole books written on what theories and models are but the most important points for me include:

1. Theory specific to midwifery (midwifery theory) is exciting because it can justify giving excellent care. You can pull theories from books to bring into your work, or find them in journals.

2. When it comes to midwifery research, instead of reinventing the wheel, researchers draw on concepts, theories and models from other disciplines like medicine and sociology. Midwifery has always used ideas from other disciplines, so an up-to-date textbook on a relevant subject will be a great help for some background reading and evidence.

(Bryar and Sinclair 2011: 29)

Once you've finished writing the main body of your essay, you can increase the reader's trust and enjoyment of your work by writing an introduction and conclusion that explains your own point of view in no uncertain terms. You can write in first person here, i.e. 'I believe that ...'.

In the introduction, you can say what you think, and what your overall opinion or answer to the question is. In your conclusion, you can say something like 'In this essay, I have explored x, which provides evidence for my belief that ...'. You don't need to do anything fancy, you just need to bring the arguments together. Use it as a way of reaffirming what kind of midwife you want to be, if at all possible. This tends to help you get your passion across which makes things more interesting as well as providing evidence of your development as a professional.

Getting critique and appraisal into your writing

At this stage, you will likely have some interesting points to make that help state the value of research or other sources you have read. It's worth thinking about how best to combine these into your writing.

Table 2.3: Getting critique and appraisal into your writing

Questions to guide your writing	Less effective	More effective
Are you using blanket statements or are you giving specific evidence and examples of what you've understood?	'Every woman or person needs kindness in their midwifery care.'	'The International Confederation of Midwives, with their global view, and the Royal College of Midwives, with their UK specific view, both mention compassion and dignity as essential components of kindness that have great relevance for midwifery care.'
Have you related your point to a midwifery theory, model, policy, or at least a concept?	'When considering screening, midwives have diverse ways of practising.'	'Different midwives might draw from the same evidence when helping clients navigate screening, but as there is no one correct overarching model of midwifery care, different models, such as the medical model and childbearing as a normal life event may be drawn on. Depending on a midwife's point of view, she might change the tone and emphasis of the information given. [reference].'
Can you say how different pieces of work or policies oppose each other?	'Midwives aiming for normality might want to concentrate on what will go well.'	'*Better Births* documented that women often feel they have to make decisions in line with what their caregiver feels is correct. However, trust policy documents often stipulate the information that each client should be offered, which by its nature might be seen as an attempt to influence a woman in a particular direction, even if midwives are focused on informed choice in care [reference].'
How does all this fit together with what you know about midwifery as a whole?	'Estimated fetal weight from scans are a way of making decisions.'	'Estimated fetal weight is one way of informing a care plan. However, the partnership model of care, which draws on the human rights act, suggests that informed choice should be the deciding factor.'
Have you offered some critique of the conclusions you have come to?	'This proves that the partnership model is one of importance in midwifery.'	'Though many midwifery organizations, guiding bodies and pieces of research cite partnership as a key aspect of the midwifery model of care, and I feel it has relevance to my clinical practice, it must be acknowledged that there was little high-level evidence involved in promoting the partnership model when it first appeared.'

A few things to consider if you're aiming for top marks. The first is that even if you come to a conclusion, you should offer some reasons why that conclusion might be incorrect. Think about how it's much easier to trust someone's point of view if you know they've considered arguments against it. The same thing applies to essay writing. Secondly, when researching this chapter I kept coming across tutors saying that a common challenge for undergraduates is finding a 'single authorial voice' (Andrews 2007). This means students get stuck converting many authors' voices into their own. Instead of a piece of writing that handles the different arguments and pieces of research in turn, students end up echoing what the researchers said, almost pretending to be them. This means writing can come across as jerky, a bit like you're becoming possessed by each author. This can make your work hard to follow, but also your tutor can lose faith in your overall argument. I think this issue is partially down to under-confidence, as it feels easier to repeat what is said by a person already established in the field. It's a way of hiding what you actually think, or not having to come to any conclusions at all.

But it's also challenging to take on so many sources and get them into a single piece of writing. Be aware of this and use the examples above, or your example essay, as a model for your writing. You should also think about your overall writing style. I don't think this has to be anything grand. Things can go wrong quickly if you crack out a thesaurus. But if reading your work is a slog, your tutor is going to end up being less persuaded by your argument because they'll lose patience. Worse than that, tutors might conclude that because your writing is hard to follow, it's likely you're confused too. To score highly, you need to write in a style that's clear and engaging.

Broad strokes style guide

The following is a list of 'Dos and Don'ts' for the writing-up stage, sourced from students and tutors. Don't feel the need to use every point but you may find one or two things that are perfect for you.

Don't:

- Spend time making sentences overly beautiful or crafted or use over-flowery language. You'll make a bigger impact if you show you've understood the subject and make a rational argument using simple language.
- Write without depth. 'Breastfeeding/chestfeeding is critically important', 'clients feel strongly about breastfeeding/ chestfeeding' should be more like 'evidence suggests

breastfeeding/chestfeeding has an irreplaceable impact on maternal/birthing person and infant bonding but there are significant validity issues with any such study as they cannot include a control group, and expert opinion repeatedly suggests that though breast/chestfeeding is the biological norm, informing clients that their relationship with their child will be harmed if they bottle-feed is both unethical and dubious [reference]'.

● If you're not able to critically analyse you probably need to go back one stage. It can be painful to realize you have to go back into research mode yet again but the odds are you're not clear on what your conclusion is yet. It's an iterative process, it's actually a great thing if you're overlapping and doubling back on your stages, it means you have a lively essay on your hands and you are engaged with it.

Do:

● Write in the third person for the main body of your essay: 'this is understood to mean ...', rather than 'I understood this to mean ...'.

● Have a look at the plagiarism policy of your university. I highly doubt anyone reading this book would knowingly plagiarize but it's vital to get this right. Essentially, anything you write that is verbatim from the source needs quote marks around it and a reference; anything you've put in your own words from a source also needs a reference. You will need to submit your work to a plagiarism checker like 'Turnitin'.

● Write the main body of your essay first, so you can make sure your introduction and conclusion fit later.

● Think criticism and analysis, rather than your own feelings or take on things.

● Use 'topic sentences'. Try and make the first sentence of each section introduce the subject matter. If possible, this sentence should also provide a link between the previous paragraph and the content of the next; for example, 'The Royal College of Midwives have also commented on the lack of resources for good postnatal care, and they add that breastfeeding ...' (Barrass 2005: 102).

● Use a basic structure to keep on task. For example, the PEE acronym stands for Point, Evidence, Explain. There are lots of different acronyms out there for essay writing but if you stick to the basic idea that you need to provide a reference and explanation for each point you make, you're on the right track.

- Express the content of the sources you've read in your own words. You can of course quote but it's usually better to show you've understood the points by writing the ideas out yourself.
- Involve all the different requirements of your essay task, there are usually marks given for balance.
- Most universities have a subscription to a referencing tool; for instance, *Cite Them Right* (Bloomsbury 2022) will help you pick up marks for correct referencing.

Things to try if you get stuck

1. Some people like those fidget toys to get rid of nervous energy while writing.
2. Have a nap. I've solved many creative and academic problems that way. Are you overtired from shift work? Naps can help.
3. Make a list of what you do know early on. Writing projects are hard because they're uncertain, it's like blowing into a balloon, the first bit is hard, the rest is easier; make a move to get started (Godin 2015).
4. If you can't seem to get going have a look at your example essay, you can't steal the first line but you can see the approach they've used and be inspired.
5. Follow your curiosity. Inspiration is a very heavy concept, but is there anything in your work that you're even a bit curious about? Follow this feeling to get into a flow state (Gilbert 2015: 68).
6. Despite what I said earlier, you may want to write your introduction first to propel you into writing. It often ends up being scaffolding, i.e. you take it away at the end as you rewrite, but it can still be helpful to get you started.
7. Make a map of quotes that you want to use in your essay and build around that.
8. Ask for specific feedback on your essays, have an appointment with a lecturer and tell them where you're getting stuck – they might have an insight you just can't see right now.
9. One person I know puts *Friends* or something else light on in the background while they're starting and eventually they get sucked into the work and turn it off. Or having a song on repeat can work too.

Basic structure

I also want to leave you with a cheat for if it all goes wrong and you run out of time. I would suggest working from the start of this chapter but if real life hits, have a go with these questions if you want. It's helped me more times than I care to admit.

Box 2.6: A basic structure

What does common sense suggest I need to include?

What are the midwifery perspectives, and what are the non-midwifery perspectives?

What are the wider social and ethical implications?

Have I covered who's most vulnerable and what can be done to protect them?

Have I added academic appraisal or critique for each of these points?

To conclude

It's worth noting that all of this stuff comes together with time and it's okay if it feels difficult to begin with. Like all skills, you'll probably start off trying to execute every element perfectly, which will take a long time. Then gut instinct will come into play and you'll be able to do things faster and know where you can half-ass it without losing marks. This is what students report, anyway.

Or you might find things straightforward because you've been well prepared by A-Levels or an Access Course, and this is fine too. You might well find it starts to get difficult sometime during the second year when things start to ramp up. Come back to review this chapter and go and see your lecturers.

The step up to degree level means independently finding new research to read, and learning new ways of interpreting, discussing and critiquing it. What you're doing isn't easy. If you're feeling awful know that setbacks and failures are part of success, as much as that sucks, it's like the bear hunt, you have to go through it!

Academic work can be stuffy and over-complicated. But at its heart, essay writing in midwifery should be about finding answers to hard decisions about childbearing. You are smart enough to figure it out. Mostly midwifery is so complicated that we just end up with better questions rather than certain answers. You're definitely capable of figuring that out. But if you have kids or a big life experience or whatever else might be going on, you might be procrastinating. The best of us do it. You'll get there. Self-compassion at all times.

Appendix

There is an example essay on midwifediaries.com that was contributed by Melissa Newman, the midwife I mentioned earlier in this chapter. Melissa is now undertaking her PhD and I've also made a video going through what she did so well. The essay is from the second year of Melissa's degree and is entitled 'Complications Around Childbirth: Pre-eclampsia Toxaemia'. It gained a First class grade (Newman 2021).

3   **Exams**

Introduction

I used to think exams were a test of intelligence, but these days I see them as more of a test of project management. We're better off doing intense bursts of revision little and often, which means the hard bit is working out how to revise around placement, assignments and other commitments. In this chapter, we'll cover revision sessions that take advantage of the physiology of learning. We'll also cover specific strategies for essay, open book and multiple choice exams, and Objective Structured Clinical Examinations (OSCEs).

How we learn

Learning is the movement of knowledge from short to long term memory. This takes physiological processes which grow and strengthen neural connections (Fields, 2020). This is hard work and feels tough for most people. Often revision will look something like reading and re-reading textbooks, but this activity is usually too easy to make the requisite changes (Brown, 2014, p.7). To make the physical changes necessary to internalize new information, you have to put your brain under the stress of trying to remember it. Revision techniques with this kind of effectiveness are all types of 'active learning', and methods include covering up your notes and trying to rewrite them, drawing out mind maps from memory, using revision cards or doing quizzes or practice tests. Later in the chapter, I'll also go into the evidence around when to revise, as spaced repetition and interleaving are both techniques which can give you a better result for the amount of effort you have put in.

What to learn

There is an almost unlimited amount of midwifery information that you could choose to learn, and therefore being discerning is key. For some topics, for example, the role of haemoglobin, it is necessary to be able to explain what is happening on a molecular level. For other topics, such as the third stage of labour, you only need to show an understanding of the anatomy and physiology and hormonal pathways involved. Before you start to revise, I would look at the type of information that has been covered in your lectures and consider how you might be tested in your exam. Ali Abdaal, a Cambridge-educated doctor who now runs a YouTube channel on studying, calls this stage of revision 'scoping out the subject' (Abdaal 2010).

To do this you should try and work out why you're studying the topic. Is it to give you knowledge that will underpin your practice as an expert in normal physiological childbearing? Or are you trying to increase your knowledge of medical conditions in pregnancy? This kind of big picture approach to considering your revision will help you make judgement calls about the most important areas to focus on (Abdaal 2020; Yonis 2020).

Before you use a revision technique

Before you start to use your revision technique, you'll need to have a good level of understanding of the topic (Abdaal 2020; Yonis 2020). If you have a suspicion that you don't understand what's going on you can check by pretending that you need to explain the topic to a child (Cunff 2020). For example, say you want to learn about the contraction of the uterus after birth and the interlacing muscle fibres known as living ligatures. I checked my understanding by writing out an explanation that I think could be understood by a ten-year-old with no prior knowledge:

> A ligature is a tool used in surgery to stop bleeding. The word comes from the Latin 'ligat' meaning 'tied'. A surgeon uses 'ligature forceps' for clamping big blood vessels during an operation. After a baby is born, the placenta, which is the organ that supplied the baby with oxygen and nutrients during pregnancy, detaches, leaving some blood vessels exposed. This is a problem because changes in pregnancy mean these blood vessels, get really 'dilated', or bigger and can carry a lot of blood. They are sometimes known as 'tortuous' or spiral because this shape helps them carry more blood. They do this so a baby can be really well supplied. The blood flow to the area can be as much as 800ml per minute. After birth, the placental bed, or the site where the placenta was, needs to be sealed off somehow. The hormone oxytocin makes a big contraction causing the uterus to become much smaller, which helps. But you also get muscles that run across the uterus pulling upwards, and the blood vessels that run through them get ligatured, and this is known as a 'living ligature'. This is the body's way of trying to get the bleeding to stop. The process is sometimes known as 'haemostasis'.

And then this write up can be used to make a revision resource.

Most of the above is from *Myles Midwifery Anatomy and Physiology Colouring Workbook* (Rankin 2014: 215). I find this kind of book helpful not so much because of the colouring but because of the many self-tests with answers. Active learning, with its self-testing focus, should start as soon as you understand the material, as opposed to waiting until a test feels comfortable (Brown 2014: 131). You can't write out this amount of detail for every term you need to cover in your revision but hopefully you can see how to teach yourself and test yourself on the harder ideas. 80/20 may well come into play here.

Active learning revision techniques

Revision cards

I like to use Anki, which is a free app for making revision cards. It's great because all I need to do a revision session is my phone. Anki will automatically present you with an optimal number of topics, based on your previous scores and optimal spaced repetition psychology research. Using Anki in the odd moment you have free on shift is a great idea given what we know about interleaving. Interleaving is where you aim to avoid feeling fluent with your revision, and so study particular areas little and often instead of doing a binge learn (for more on this, see later in this chapter). Having a revision resource that is indexable can also make revision cards double as a useful way of looking up information when you're in clinical practice.

Mind maps

You can use mind maps to revise as recreating these without looking at the original material is another way of self-testing. Students talk about mind maps offering useful visual reminders. It seems to be a very stimulating form of revision for people who enjoy visual resources (Yonis 2021). You might already know about the utterly beautiful mind maps and diagrams that can be found online at the Student Midwife Studygram (studentmidwifestudygram.co.uk) (no affiliation).

Highlighting

Most education researchers say that highlighting and underlining does little to aid learning (Abdaal 2020; Brown 2014; Yonis 2021). I suspect students who use this method and get good results are also self-testing, for instance identifying clusters of ideas and keywords, and writing out bullet points or short summaries.

Covering up the textbook or notes

A simple way to revise is to cover up your textbook or notes and quiz yourself on the content. I find it tricky to remember what I should be asking myself but with practice I bet this is a solid revision technique. One advantage is you don't have to spend extra time making revision cards or other materials.

Mnemonic systems

Mnemonic systems use a pattern of letters, ideas or some other easy way to remember something. They can be extremely useful. A common one for remembering what to auscultate while performing a cardiovascular examination on a newborn is 'All Prostitutes Take Money':

Aortic

Pulmonary

Tricuspid

Mitral

(Anon 2012).

There are a few useful mnemonics you will come across during your course; for instance, '4 is the floor' for remembering that a blood glucose level of less than 4 mmol/l is hypoglycemia (i.e. the patient will end up on the floor soon). There's another for the spelling of diarrhoea: 'Dash In A Real Rush, Hurry Or Else Accident'. I love a good mnemonic, and they are a part of midwifery/medical culture, but you probably won't be able to come up with one for everything you need to remember.

Memory palace

With a 'memory palace', the idea is to assign a topic to a physical space, like a coffee shop or study area of the library you know well.

To quote from the teaching YouTube channel 'Sprouts' (2017):

Imagine some sort of familiar physical space, like your house, school or office, and then add a mental image of the thing you want to remember. To remember a bunch of things you can use different rooms and visualise how you would walk through that space following the same specific route. As you walk through, place the things you want to remember at specific locations, ideally, imagining things in a funny or crazy way.

I've used this technique for particularly slippery information that I couldn't get to stick, and it can be a good excuse to revise somewhere nice so you have different spaces to draw on (pubs during the day are usually quieter than coffee shops, making them a useful place to revise in general, and this technique should come easily in them) (Brown 2014: 184).

Interleaving

Interleaving means switching between subjects as you revise as there is evidence to suggest this is more effective than 'massed practice' (Brown 2014: 149). When I was revising for my GCSEs I'd spend a whole morning on one subject before switching to a different subject in the afternoon. It was comfortable. However, the next day I'd find I'd forgotten a lot of what I'd covered and would have to start all over again. If this feels like a familiar story, you might want to revise one topic for, say, no more than an hour before starting a new one. For instance, if you use revision cards to work on infant feeding for an hour, you're best off switching to blood groups or another topic for the next hour. In the short term, this will feel harder but your overall progress will be faster. Some experts suggest you should study a topic for no more than twenty minutes. Others suggest you should study for long enough to have a sense of accomplishment, as you should try not to use interleaving as a way of avoiding a topic that's hard (Weinstein 2016).

Spaced repetition

Spaced repetition is a similar idea to interleaving but takes advantage of psychology research that suggests there is an optimal timing pattern for learning. Say you have a new set of revision cards, have a look at the table below for a suggested schedule. I've tried this, it really works, with the obvious proviso that it has to be content which you found easy to study on the first session. For more challenging material, spaced repetition is useful but you may have to attempt 'day 1' a few times before implementing spaced repetition is possible.

Table 3.1: Spaced repetition study sessions

Day 1	1st study session
Day 2	2nd study session
Day 7	3rd study session
Day 30	4th study session
Day 60	5th study session

(Young 2021)

Revision timetables

Because some topics are harder than others and will require more time spent on them, I don't find a traditional study timetable to be very useful. Instead, you need a living document that you can adapt as the challenges in your revision become clearer.

I make a spreadsheet of topics that could come up, and after every revision session I add the date I revised and then colour code it green, amber or red depending on how I did. I can then see which topics are in need of most work. This is another Ali Abdaal suggestion (2010). It works well because if you find a subject challenging, you don't have to panic, you can just adapt your study plans to include more time spent on it.

Table 3.2: Traffic light revision timetable

Pre-eclampsia	1/9/21	12/9/21	18/9/21
Fetal development	1/9/21	1/9/21	25/9/21
Cardiovascular system	11/9/21	1/9/21	25/9/21
Drug calculations	11/9/21	13/9/21	25/9/21

Strategies for specific types of exam

1 Essay exams

Revision

What you write in an essay during a timed exam will differ from what you can include in an assignment that you have weeks to complete. Typically, written exams will test your knowledge of anatomy and physiology and/or key clinical skills and most of what you mention will be purely factual and based on what you've been taught in lectures. If you have a closed-book exam, where you're not able to take any resources in with you, you will likely need to rote learn some references to use in your answers.

A strategy to revise for these exams might be:

1. Look at the topics covered in lectures and brainstorm ideas for practice questions.
2. Look at a mark scheme if you have one.
3. Use a textbook or midwifery handbook to find key information that you can use to answer the practice questions.

4. Choose references to learn. Useful references that can be used in lots of different essay answers include a midwifery textbook; a professional code; a recent report that summarizes the main mortality and morbidity risks; an important guideline; a piece of research about the midwifery model of care; any piece of high-quality evidence that you are passionate about.

5. Use this information to implement active learning memorization tools like revision cards, mind maps, etc.

Structure

When writing timed essays under pressure, the hardest thing for me is structure, and from talking to students it sounds like this is a common challenge.

There are different ways of structuring an essay answer.

- Some students like to aim for an introduction, then three main paragraphs and a conclusion, which is a simple way of doing things. This might work perfectly for some questions, but for others, it could create an essay that is too short or is difficult to follow as you have to arbitrarily group ideas into three categories.

- Some students start with the simplest points and build in complexity, so for instance, starting with basic anatomy and physiology knowledge and building toward applying that to comment on how care is organized.

- Ali Abdaal suggests writing an introduction that summarizes the main argument of your essay, and then continuing your introduction by stating key parts of your argument in numbered points, '(1), (2), (3)', etc. You can then go on to number your paragraphs (1), (2), (3), etc. which makes for a tidy, easy-to-follow format (Abdaal 2019).

- I have four prompts which help me structure my thoughts.

- My basic areas to cover are:

    1. Common sense
    2. Midwifery responsibilities
    3. The wider social and ethical considerations
    4. Protecting the most vulnerable clients.

An example of how I might use this structure is below.

Table 3.3: Essay plan for exam question: *Describe the midwife's role in postnatal care in normal healthy childbearing concentrating on anatomy and physiology returning to the pre-pregnant state.*

Essay prompt	Points to include	Books/ resources to reference
Common sense: in this case, I would take this to mean the anatomy and physiology knowledge I have	Breasts/chest anatomy and breastfeeding/chestfeeding Uterine involution and lochia The healing of 1st and 2nd degree tears Passing urine Bowel movements Mobilization and returning to exercise Mental well-being	Skills for Midwifery Practice Midwife Labour and Birth Handbook NMC Code NICE postnatal guidelines
Midwifery responsibilities	Immediate postnatal period, i.e. after 3rd stage of labour; observations, blood loss, bladder care, return to normal hydration and nutrition, rh negative blood type Postnatal care at home: as above, pelvic floor exercises Usually care for 10 days but up to 6 weeks Handing care to the health visitor Care of the newborn is out of remit but briefly mention this as critical part of midwifery care	Skills for Midwifery Practice Midwife Labour and Birth Handbook NMC Code NICE postnatal guidelines
The wider social and ethical considerations	Do women or pregnant people actually return to their non-pregnant state? Society expectations about weight gain/ stretch marks, breastfeeding/ chestfeeding continuing and mental change of parenthood	Midwife Labour and Birth Handbook
Protecting the most vulnerable clients	Informed choice; do we truly offer this? Women and birthing people should not think the following are normal and 'put up' with them: Urinary incontinence, Dyspareunia Blood loss; melanated skin staff lack ability to assess colour May lack expertise on transgender and non-binary care in terms of what is normal for breast/chestfeeding	NHS Resolution Montgomery Report MBRRACE Workshop on safe LGBTQIA+ midwifery care

Timing

The amount of time you spend writing your answer will differ depending on the exam length, but the following is a good guide if, for example, you had a ninety-minute exam in which you were required to write two answers.

Box 3.1: Approximate timings allocated in a written exam of 90 minutes

Q1: 10 minutes planning, 25 minutes writing, 5 minutes checking through

Q2: 10 minutes planning, 25 minutes writing, 5 minutes checking through

10 minutes of extra time allocated as necessary

For a typical undergraduate midwifery exam, most of my word count would be spent on the top two boxes in the table above, and I'd aim to use the rest for rounding things off in a client-centred way.

Technique

The following ideas may be helpful in handwriting your answers.

- Using less than (<) or more than (>) symbols can help reduce the number of words you have to write out (a useful way of remembering these is < looks most like an 'l' for less than).
- Use numerals when writing amounts or other numbers.
- Writing out the full name for something, for example, Nursing and Midwifery Council (NMC), the first time you use it is best practice, though you can use the abbreviation after that.
- Almost no one will be perfect with spelling and grammar under time pressure but it's worth checking through afterwards.
- My instincts are to write as fast as possible, but actually in the practice questions I completed in writing this book, my work where I've slowed down has been of better quality and more legible.

Practice

Students differ in the amount they write and the only way of truly working out your game plan is by trying some questions under exam conditions. You can't do this for every possible question, but if we use the 80/20 rule again (which says that 80 per cent of your ability will come from 20 per cent of your revision), you might be able to make an educated guess about the questions that are most likely to come up and practise those essays in full (Tanabe 2018). For questions that seem less likely to come up, just practise putting together an essay plan.

2   Open-book exams

If it's an open-book exam the material you cover might be more complex. I would still scope out a list of practice questions and follow the steps above in working out the reasons for the exam and the level of detail you think is necessary, but you can add some more complicated or wider social and ethical insights. For instance, you might comment on the type of research or a particular model or theory and how it applies to the question. In the postnatal care question above I might talk about the salutogenic approach providing a balance to the current emphasis on medicalized care, and how this might be used in normal healthy childbearing.

The rest of your preparation will be similar to that required for other written exams, but instead of memorizing points and references, bookmark relevant pages or make useful summary notes to take in with you. Make index cards with bullet points of useful information and references. You could also take in your lecture notes or mind maps, depending on your preference. Finally, have a go at making essay structures and writing out a few answers in full using your practice questions. You're aiming to be familiar with your resources to the point that it's quick and simple to slot together an essay structure, so you can spend the majority of your time writing (Simon Fraser University, 2013).

3   Multiple choice exams

When it comes to answering multiple choice questions one technique is to read the question while covering up the possible answers. In this way, you can work with what you know rather than being impacted by the choices (Richardson 2020). I would try and find past papers and practise with these.

I would also use my lecture notes, syllabus and a textbook to make an educated guess about the topics that could come up. The amount of information you need to revise is likely to be greater than that for written exams because multiple choice papers can cover a lot of topics (Richardson 2020)

As you know, I use Anki revision cards. If I were revising for a multiple choice exam I would share my cards with a few other students. Hopefully, they would share their revision resources with me and together we could make sure we'd covered all the needed topics.

4 Objective Structured Clinical Examinations

Objective Structured Clinical Examinations (OSCEs) are used on midwifery courses to test your practical skills. In the early part of your training, you might get tested on routine skills like abdominal palpation, venepuncture or intramuscular injection. As you progress through your course, OSCEs could cover emergencies or other complex situations.

In practical exams, you will need to provide answers quickly as you are speaking rather than writing. Hopefully, you will have revised enough for the basics to become easy to describe. However, you're not looking for a careful critical analysis and questioning of practice, you just need to demonstrate:

- that you are a safe professional, who routinely performs basics like hand hygiene and universal precautions, such as wearing an apron and gloves;
- that your client understands what's happening, you offer information so they can consent (or not) and you form good rapport;
- that you can perform a clinical task;
- that you can explain why the clinical task is needed, and your rationale is clear;
- that you explain your findings back to the client and tell them about any next steps;
- that you document your actions clearly.

(Bloomfield et al. 2010: 61; Medistudents 2021)

You'll want to make a list of all possible scenarios, and then learn responses from trusted sources to address those scenarios. Many of these will be covered in an essential skills book, or as you progress through your course, in a handbook of obstetric emergencies. It's best to find one that is recommended by your course and is relevant to your country. For instance in the UK at the time of writing, most students will use the Prompt guide for revising for their final-year OSCEs (Winter et al. 2018). Some people write out a whole script and learn it verbatim or break down responses onto revision cards.

When committing your answers to memory, don't neglect your essential midwifery care skills. Remember the basics like introducing yourself, and privacy and dignity. To take the example of talking through how you'd do a vaginal examination, ask if the client wants to void their bladder beforehand and remember to auscultate the fetal heart both before and after the procedure. Document your findings, making sure the date and your name are clear.

If you're very overwhelmed and there seems to be too much information to learn, look for the top 20 per cent of information to revise (Tanabe 2018). You can also look at mark schemes, though have a go at answering before you look at these, it's a great opportunity to start using active recall, which is what will commit the detail to long-term memory. It also might be useful to think about the theatre needed to perform well at an OSCE. Many students record themselves answering OSCE questions and watch the recording to mark it. Revising with your peers can be very helpful for this reason, as marking other performances can give you an idea of what it's like to be the examiner and having a go yourself can replicate exam conditions. It can also help you get over initial stage fright and awkwardness as you try and pretend you're actually in practice.

Plenty of brilliant midwives struggle with OSCEs. It's hard because it's a test of what you know about the guidelines and policies first and foremost. We know there are changes that need to be made in midwifery but you can't do activism at the same time as passing an OSCE, or at least it's hard to make this your main focus (although one day I'd love to see an activism OSCE, wouldn't you?)

You may also have an OSCE as an end of programme assessment that could cover any topic covered in your training. These are sometimes set up as a conversation, rather than being about practical skill and might be known as a 'viva voce' exam, which means 'living voice' in Latin (Gale Group 2008). The point will be to talk the examiner through a safe care plan. This is a tricky type of exam to prepare for because you could get something that you haven't covered for a while. The ideal would be to have revision cards or another active recall method that you have built up during your training which you review again, but I can't say I managed to be that organized during my degree. Otherwise, I would work with a midwifery textbook that you know well and do peer support study sessions where you ask each other questions in test conditions.

It also might be useful to take a step back and look at your training as a whole, and ask why this final OSCE or Viva exists. We can see it's a capstone exam and it's about you being ready to join the register and take a position as a newly qualified midwife. Therefore it's probably not going to be on academic knowledge alone and won't be about getting you to describe a type of research, learning model or current report, etc. It's also not going to be on something basic like catheterization because if you can't do that kind of skill it should have been picked up earlier in your training. I would suggest what's left is obstetric emergencies, a midwife's role in looking after clients with medical conditions or solving difficult clinical leadership scenarios. Additionally, it's likely to be a somewhat urgent situation because otherwise an undeniably sensible response might be along the lines of 'I'd look it up in the guidelines' or 'I'd refer them to a midwifery/medical specialist' and this wouldn't showcase your skills. With this in mind, I might make a list of possible questions and then use the 80/20 rule to focus on learning answers to the most likely scenarios (Tanabe 2018). For instance, talking through what you'd do if you had concerns but couldn't get a doctor to review is the kind of question that might come up. It takes a certain kind of confidence to allow yourself to think in this way, you're aiming for empathy with the tutors putting the course together. This kind of resourcefulness and problem solving can be a very useful part of exam technique.

If you do have an OSCE on obstetric emergencies, there are several good YouTube videos by an organization called Health E-Learning and Media (2018). I particularly like their mnemonic 'SOAPs' for remembering the staff you need to summon during an emergency: Senior Midwives, Obstetrician, Anaesthetist, Paediatrician.

Motivation for revision

Motivation is something that comes in seasons. I also think it's hard to find the motivation to revise if you have many competing priorities. If you're feeling under pressure but also a bit burnt out, have a look at the following tips.

1. Sometimes it helps to focus on learning the information you need to be a good midwife and be able to serve your clients well.

2. In my experience people enjoy being around someone who is revising, we like to see people with a purpose. Perhaps get your partner or kids to quiz you (if the material is age-appropriate) or even start a YouTube channel. Teaching is the ultimate way of checking you understand.

3. Sleep really helps with learning. I've referred to the physical changes that strengthen the connections between neurons. If you start an intense new exercise regime, recovery including sleep is essential for your body to get stronger. In the same way, sleep supports you with exam technique (Walker and van der Helm

2009). I know you might be struggling to get enough rest, but if you can tweak your revision period to include more sleep, you're probably going to see better results (and enjoy it more too).

4. If you don't feel like you're coping, it's worth going to the library/student services and asking for a one-to-one session. Be really honest about what's going on. If this service isn't available, look for an independent tutor. I know not everyone can afford it, but doing just a couple of sessions can help. If you are struggling it's likely you need a hand transferring your own particular brand of intelligence into an exam-friendly format. It will have nothing to do with how smart you are.

Tips for if you run out of time

Lots of students find themselves in the position of feeling unprepared for an exam. If this is you, perhaps see it as an opportunity to practise your improvisation skills. Improvising is something all midwives have to be good at – think about an un-booked client who comes in pushing, we have to think on our feet!

For example, say you're studying for a final-year OSCE which is on obstetric emergencies and you have a limited timeframe to revise. I might:

1. Prioritize revision topics. My go-to list of obstetric emergencies is from the UK 'Prompt' guide which includes rare events like uterine inversion and maternal cardiac arrest. Instead of starting off revising for the most unusual emergencies, I might choose to look at the more common ones, such as shoulder dystocia, postpartum haemorrhage and newborn resuscitation. It's more likely these will come up on the exam. The added benefit of starting with these is that the information you memorize will likely apply to more uncommon scenarios; for example, newborn resuscitation is a key skill for anyone attending a breech birth.

2. I might then come back to 'What questions would I be most unhappy to see if the exam were tomorrow?' This might mean manoeuvres for breech birth, positions for cord prolapse and the samples we need to take for sepsis. Revise the most critical elements and you might be surprised at how much else falls into place.

3. I might then have a go at sample OSCE questions to mark my work. If I didn't have sample questions I would make some up.

To conclude

When I was training, I liked to take a lot of time over my midwifery learning, finding tangents, extra information and many different points of view. If you're similar to me, please know that this is a strength but to prepare for exams you might want to temper your way of doing things with good planning so you can map out and memorise what's needed. Whatever your approach, you might find the idea of 'type two fun' to be helpful. Type two fun is the kind of experience that's hard graft or a bit scary while it's happening but fun to look back on as a job well done.

Presentations

Introduction

Preparing a presentation is similar to writing an essay in that the process gets you to consider deeply a topic while drawing on reliable evidence. Also like an essay, your grade will be given based on the knowledge and insight you demonstrate, and the structure behind your work. But you will also gain marks based on your visual aids, and your ability to use voice and body language to help your audience understand what you're saying. Part of presenting means delivering in an interesting and active way. It's a live medium, meaning you may need to adjust what you're saying quickly and calmly, depending on questions asked or in order to react to other presenters who go before you (University of Bangor 2021).

In this chapter, there are ideas to help you cover what is important academically. In addition, I know that public speaking is something many excellent students and midwives aren't keen on so I have also included some suggestions to help with nerves. If you want a more detailed approach to using resources and including critical analysis, you may want to review Chapter Two, which covers essays.

Getting started

A sensible path through preparing for a presentation looks something like the following.

> **Assess Presentation Task > Read Material > Critique Material > Structure Outline > Make Visual Aids > Make Prompts for Presenting > Rehearse**

But just like with any other assignment task, you will move and move back and forth through the process as you want to make changes or add more ideas.

Assessing the presentation task

When you are given your presentation title or brief, you might want to spend some time understanding exactly what you're being asked to do. Make sure you understand the question or presentation topic you are given. Identify the keywords and unpack their meaning, making notes on your findings. Look at the mark scheme and any example presentations your university has provided. Try to understand the point of this task: what do you think your tutors want you to achieve and demonstrate? If you can empathize with whoever's marking you, you're a long way to getting a good grade.

Reading the material

You may want to read Chapter Two on essays, as the process of finding resources will be similar.

In short:

- You could start by getting a general overview from resources mentioned in the reading list.
- You could then read relevant, recent articles from peer-reviewed journals or other reputable sources, especially high-quality evidence such as meta-analysis.
- You might want to check regulatory body, government and trust guidelines for other relevant information.

To give a specific example of the amount of reading I would do for a 15-minute undergraduate presentation, I might cover something like: the useful parts of a few books, five–ten peer-reviewed articles or studies, and a guideline. While reading, I would make a note of the ideas I wanted to include in my presentation, along with the reference.

Critiquing the material

Just like with essay assignments, the big marks will be available if you've covered the basics and then head towards more complex material. Covering complexity is always going to be a little risky as there's a chance you haven't fully understood or you're missing some key considerations because you're new to the field. Remember that point from Chapter Two: though you might be a small fish in a big pond, your tutors will like it if you're a brave one.

If you are in your final year, you will be expected to cover some detailed research appraisal or other assessment of the reliability of your sources. Perhaps look at Chapter Six, Engaging with research, for more.

Structuring your presentation

I tend to plan the main body of a presentation before the introduction and conclusion as I find this easiest, but there are other ways that you may find are best for you.

The following will give you an idea of what you're aiming for.

Box 4.1: Approximate structure for a 15-minute presentation

Introduction: 300 words

Main Body: 1,500 words total

> Point 1 (300 words)
>
> Point 2 (300 words)
>
> Point 3 (300 words)
>
> Point 4 (300 words)
>
> Point 5 (300 words)

Conclusion: 300 words

Have a go at splitting your ideas into a structure like Box 4.1 and know that you can always cut down further as you start to rehearse and see if your presentation is within time limits. Most sources say you should aim for 130–160 words per minute, so for a 15-minute presentation, that's just over 2,000 words in total. If we split that into a number of points that feels reasonable, it works out to something like six points overall, at 300 words each. Of course, your plan shouldn't be overly prescriptive, I don't find making a transcript very helpful, and you won't be counting words. But you'll probably be familiar with the amount of detail that a 2,000-word essay involves, so hopefully this gives you a rough idea of what you're aiming for (University of Kent 2022).

When you have a good idea of what the main body of your presentation will contain, you might want to plan your introduction and conclusion. I tend to start with these so I know what my points are following on from and building towards.

Your introduction

The purpose of your introduction is to help your audience understand the scope of the topic at hand and the specific ideas and direction your presentation will include. The introduction to a presentation should also engage the audience, so perhaps use a video clip, a powerful image or a story from practice (though remember to keep things confidential).

Your conclusion

All you need to do with a conclusion is to remind the audience of what they've learnt, the main argument and the evidence you cited. Sometimes at the end of a presentation, it's good to mention one thing the audience should walk away with, which might be a little-known fact or an evidence-based change for their midwifery practice. You can then invite questions from the audience.

Starting to rehearse

Moving from a structure or plan of a presentation to being able to actually deliver it might mean working through a few awkward attempts where you don't know what you're doing yet. I think many of us spend time in this intermediate stage and I actually like to increase the pressure by videoing myself, as it helps me imagine there is an audience watching. This helps me identify where I need to make changes, and make a few cue cards so I remember what works and what doesn't. It's also a great way of starting to practise the material and to make creative connections between ideas that don't at first seem to have any link.

However, some people want to make all of their cue cards/notes, and design their PowerPoint/visual aids before having a run-through. Go with what works for you but the downside to this option is that you may need to go back and make some changes (not that this is the end of the world).

PowerPoint

I've read that PowerPoint was invented by a person with dyslexia (Hargreaves 2016: 146) and I can see that being true. When it's used well, PowerPoint can show clear links between concepts, and introduce just a few select ideas at a time. Your university library might have a PowerPoint guide, so perhaps check their website.

The following are some ideas to help you use PowerPoint:

- You can use speaker notes that are visible on your monitor, but are not visible to the audience. I've always found it a bit too difficult to use these; I prefer physical cue cards, but you may find the notes option to be perfect for you.

- Remember you'll need to go further than just reading your slides to access high marks.

- Don't include too many fancy features. Go for colours that are consistent and not too crowded or loud. Most software you'll be using will have example presentations you can adapt, or if you are building a presentation around a particular graph, perhaps choose your colour theme based on what it contains.

- Slides can turn people off so try and be immediately interesting. As mentioned above, an anecdote or even a short video can be a great way to begin; the use of storytelling as a way of learning in healthcare is well documented (Gould 2017).

As you know, you don't have to use PowerPoint. Sometimes the best way of holding attention is to make your presentation about verbal communication first and foremost. I've done several presentations using cue cards and just two PowerPoint slides which were infographics. The only time I used slides was to show diagrams for concepts that could not be explained with language alone.

Visuals

Other options apart from PowerPoint include a visual aid on a white-board or flipchart which you can annotate, or something that you print onto handouts, so everyone in your class gets a copy. The images you use should add to what you say rather than lead it. Use easy-to-under-stand diagrams, and perhaps graphs as long as you help the audience interpret them. Don't overuse visuals as this can make things hard for your audience to follow.

Reasons you might want to use an image include:

- to introduce your presentation and main argument or concept
- to introduce the structure of your presentation and help achieve flow
- to provide definitions of keywords or concepts
- to highlight main or new points
- to pull together the ideas to a succinct conclusion.

Guidance on images:

- each image should be easily understandable
- make the text and diagrams clear and readable
- keep your images consistent (use the same font, titles, layout, etc., for each image)

- make sure your images are of high quality (check for spelling and other errors)
- it can also be a good idea to include a slide that shows connections between ideas or concepts, as this demonstrates integration in your thinking.

(University of Leicester 2020)

Group presentations

For group presentations, you'll probably need to each choose an area of the assignment to concentrate on, and then bring it all together to rehearse. Having some ground rules is a great idea but how you bring this up will depend on group dynamics. Sometimes group work is a bit of an exercise in compromise, which is a key midwifery skill; teamwork and communication are parts of the task.

Try to have smooth transitions between group members; link the ideas together by saying 'Well as Keelie was saying, screening information is received by clients in different ways, and to explore further ...'.

If appropriate there might be time for a short role-play which can be an engaging method of demonstrating a concept and therefore picking up marks. Having an idea of what to say if one group member doesn't attend is a good idea; perhaps everyone could have a copy of each other's notes.

Delivery and nervousness

It's not unusual to feel nervous about public speaking. Being able to communicate well to a group is an essential skill for midwives (think leading antenatal classes) but it can seem a bit unfair if you feel you won't do well during presentations but everything else in your clinical and university work is going well.

I've presented at quite a few conferences and often feel out of my depth, especially when I'm sharing a stage with professionals with many years of experience or far higher academic credentials. There are a few ideas I come back to. The first is one I also use in practice a lot. When I'm scared of what's happening, I visualize a torch in my hand and imagine it represents my attention. I then choose to shine it out to the client I'm caring for instead of on myself. You can do this during a presentation by shining your attention onto the information you're sharing and the reaction of your audience.

Another concept that might be helpful is something I learned from a writing mentor of mine. She described the concept of 'push communicators' and 'pull communicators'. Push communicators are people who find it easy to share their thoughts. In contrast, pull communicators do a lot of thinking behind the scenes. They often feel 'Why would anyone want to hear from me?' and only share their suggestions if asked directly. These types of people are often brilliant at holding space during a birth. Sometimes I wonder if student midwives and midwives who don't enjoy presenting are pull communicators and by asking them to stand up in a room full of people, we're asking them to change their nature. If you're in this category and find presentations hard, I'd say that my experience in writing groups with pull communicators is that their work is thoughtful, interesting and has been considered from many angles. Sometimes it's about letting people in to see your work, so you might have to be generous on this occasion; this is something I learned from the writer Megan Macedo.

The one factor that I believe helps most of us is to practise enough times that the content becomes easy to talk through (Hargreaves 2016: 22). Most of us speak too quickly during presentations, so make a conscious effort to slow down. Keep your message and language simple. Speak clearly, but don't change your personality or word choice too much; you do need to communicate as yourself, just stick to the professional version of yourself. In my experience you're unlikely to achieve all this by reading out a transcript word by word; some of it has to be at least a little bit improvised.

Another technique is from Michael Grinder, a public speaking expert, who suggests the 'cat-dog' model. Under pressure, some of us can communicate quickly, be eager to please and be friendly. But gravitas in public speaking often comes from commanding the room, slowing our speech down and considering what others are saying, like a cat surveying things but remaining emotionally unengaged. Grinder suggests that the more reactive method of communication is a bit dog-like and the less reactive method is more cat-like. If you want to command a room, you may find leaning into a more cat-like mode may help (Grinder, in Goyder 2014: 234). I don't know if this is an evidence-based trick but I've used it at times with good effect. I've also used music on my phone before speaking at conferences, sometimes calming stuff, sometimes something more positive and mood-enhancing.

You may also want to try rehearsing by videoing yourself. You can then pick out the moments when you're communicating best and then do more of that. This is a good confidence-building activity, even though it's always a bit cringey watching ourselves back. It's also a great way of checking timing, though don't be surprised if you find you have to shorten your presentation by compressing ideas. Cutting things down can turn your presentation into a bit of a mess which can be very demoralizing but every time I've had to do this, I've made it work in the end and the presentation has been leaner, more on point and more engaging.

If you're watching your presentation back and think it's a bit confusing, perhaps try adding a topic sentence at the beginning of each segment to signpost what's going to happen next. For instance 'For the following reasons, many midwives prefer to talk about "chance" as opposed to "risk" when discussing screening ...'. Even better are topic sentences that link concepts or segments together; for example, 'We've covered the mathematical concepts that come with describing risk, however, for the following reasons, many midwives prefer to talk about "chance" as opposed to risk ...'.

I have a terrible time pronouncing professional terms. It took me until halfway through my training to stop saying 'perennial' instead of 'perineal' and I'm pretty sure there are loads of mispronunciations on my YouTube channel. Try and listen to words you haven't come across in a video and write them out phonetically, and if there is a cultural difference involving someone's name or another important word, it's even more important to pronounce that correctly (Xango 2017). However, if you do get something wrong, and are corrected, apologize calmly and move on. We've all been there and tutors and others watching you learning in action is a good thing.

Try and anticipate some of the questions you might get asked so you can have some answers prepared. If you don't know the answer to one of the questions that get asked you could say you'll look into it, and you could also ask your lecturer if they know. Adding that you can email round your PowerPoint/some notes and the references is a nice touch and shows you're good at teaching.

Dress suitably – the usual advice is for smart office wear. I guess wear something that makes you feel confident and professional. Having some bottled water with one of those sports tops is a good idea; I don't know how I've got to my age without learning that drinking and breathing are different activities, but I find a sports top helps me not to choke, especially if I'm under pressure.

You might have to find workarounds depending on your strengths and weaknesses; for example I know some of my dyslexic friends hate writing on a whiteboard because having to spell in front of an audience is a nightmare, but PowerPoint presentations or videos make things simple.

Along with recording your presentation performance and watching it back, another very useful strategy is to find another student midwife online to present to and then ask for feedback. You can often find someone via a Facebook group or on Instagram and the process should help both of you learn. I know this can feel a bit like hard work but I've done this several times and the constructive criticism, and the practice of presenting in real conditions, can make a huge difference.

I'm not sure that I will have solved 100 per cent of the problems so it's worth pointing out that if your presentation is dominating your life and making you really anxious, a trip to the GP might be in order. In my experience, there are many brilliant people out there who are strong and resilient but who simply aren't getting the support they need.

Other types of presentation

Poster presentations

You might be set an assignment that includes making a poster and giving a short presentation about it. Posters are usually large, bright and informative. They are designed to catch people's attention at conferences, where the aim is to share research and network. They are often centred around the image or graphic. Your university might have a bank of template posters for you to have a look at.

You should put your text into columns or grids that read left to right; a style we're familiar with from newspapers or magazines. I'd think about including six–ten key parts of a poster for a 15-minute presentation (Staffordshire University 2017) – have a look at the following example.

Waterbirth

Waterbirth in Wider Context of Midwifery – Some Background and a Key Argument for Use

Here you might write an introduction to the topic, include reliable evidence (200–300 words)

What is Waterbirth?

- Guidelines around waterbirth (200 words)
- A basic overview of waterbirth in the different stages of labour
- Choice around waterbirth
- What happens in obstetric emergency

The Physiology of the Woman/Birthing Person in Water

(200 words)
- Explanation [reference]
- Explanation [reference]

(200 words)

Explanation [reference]
Explanation [reference]
Explanation [reference]

Waterbirth and Labour

- Guidelines around waterbirth (200 words)
- A basic overview of waterbirth in the different stages of labour
- Choice around waterbirth
- What happens in obstetric emergency

Infographic/graph/table which explores the evidence around waterbirth, either one from a high-quality piece of research (check your trust guidelines) or one you have created yourself

Remember to reference or self-credit

Waterbirth and the Midwife's Role

(400 words)
- Point, Evidence, Explain [reference]
- Point, Evidence, Explain [reference]
- Point, Evidence, Explain [reference]
- Point, Evidence, Explain [reference]

Conclusion

(200 words)
- Point, Evidence, Explain [reference]
- Point, Evidence, Explain [reference]

References

Harvard reference list (it's acceptable to use a smaller font to get these on)

Your portfolio

I see a portfolio as a kind of presentation of your work, albeit a paper one. When someone looks through your portfolio they should be able to see what you have to offer as a professional, and the kind of learning, reflection and client care you have undertaken. It's a bird's eye view of what you've done and how far you've come.

Student portfolios will contain professional learning plans, relevant assignments, reflections (many courses will get you to write extra reflections as part of your portfolio that aren't necessarily graded), details about drug learning, cards or letters from clients as evidence of your care, action plans, practice hours, drug calculation tests, certificates from study days, courses or conferences and anything else you think is useful. Your university should give you guidelines for your portfolio. For me at least, a portfolio is an exercise in collecting information, putting it in an easy-to-follow order, and then choosing some reflections and case studies to include.

I think some of us feel a little awkward about portfolios because the point is to capture you mid-learning, so some pieces of writing or learning outcomes will be less accomplished than others. Rather than trying to show off, use it as almost a diary of your progress (though everything does have to be professional and protect the confidentiality of clients).

When your university starts to introduce the idea of a portfolio and tells you what should go in it, set up a folder on your computer where you can keep portfolio items, or you may be instructed to use an electronic tool such as 'Pebble Pad'. I would also have a physical file to keep track of paper documents. As I hinted at in Chapter One, I was terrible at this as a student but have since discovered David Allen's book *Getting Things Done* (2015) which has been a huge help in becoming organized.

You might need to bring your portfolio to interviews, so any evidence of extracurricular activities like organizing a conference, being part of midwifery society or getting involved in leading study sessions are great to include and can help you with getting employment. Later in your career, you might build a portfolio around applying for a specific job role, for example, if you're applying to be a diabetes specialist midwife, you might get involved in updating trust guidelines and include those as evidence. You might remove other bits and pieces that are less relevant.

Just like with placement documents, it's worth taking photos of everything that's on paper, so if you lose something, you have a back-up.

Some insights from students

> Our university isn't too formal about having [a portfolio], it's just manda-
> tory training evidence handed in, really. I keep my own records of
> progress and compliments etc ... I just recommend that you don't leave it
> all until the end of the year!

Amy Walker

> I am now in my second year and I love having a space where I can collate
> all of my learning and development. I ... [can] identify areas for improve-
> ment or self-study. My portfolio has varying resources, from videos and
> PDFs, to scanned notes and certificates of learning. I also like to keep my
> reflective writing together ... to review how I have improved. I add any
> additional courses or sessions I have attended ... Add any resource that
> you enjoy, anything that doesn't seem like a chore and is something to
> look forward to. Be creative and show your development.

Katie McKenna

> I find the portfolio so satisfying, it's not only proof of your consolidation,
> but of your progress – and seeing it all laid out reminds you why you go
> in every day, why you do that third night shift, why you're in the library till
> 2am.

Bee Hemmings

To conclude

I've found that good presenting is usually to do with finding an angle that
you're truly interested in and a story you want to tell. If you're captivated
by what you're talking about, then your audience will be too, and you'll
likely forget about your nerves. That and being familiar with the content,
or at least being up for improvising, have been the key factors in my own
ability to present, even if I have strong feelings of nervousness.

On the other hand, I wasn't necessarily lit up for every presentation
I had to do at university. If you're lacking energy for the task you've
been set, have a think about 80/20, i.e. what is the top 20 per cent of
the content you need to cover – the best of us sometimes have to just
get it done.

5 Reflections

Introduction

Reflections are an effort to unite theory and practise by thoughtfully considering your care. When you write a reflection you think about what you know and what you don't know, and try to identify some useful lessons. Lots of midwifery students I've come across say they don't really get the point of reflections, and I suspect this is partly because when writing a reflection you have to force a complex situation onto a page, and despite our best efforts the conclusions reached can feel naive. We feel this instinctively but it's difficult to do anything about the fact that reflections are an armchair exercise.

However, despite the limitations, they are powerful pieces of work. I think of reflections almost like doing qualitative research on myself. I become a small case study and use the lens of a particular situation to work out how I can improve my practice. In this chapter, we'll explore how to get started with reflective assignments, but also how to use reflections as a learning technique that supports you.

Forms of reflective cycle

Professor Graham Gibbs of Gibbs Reflective Cycle fame is, amongst other things, a noted qualitative researcher who is interested in teaching and learning. He has a great YouTube channel that includes some of his lectures, and you might understand the context of reflections better if you have a look at it (Gibbs 2010). Essentially, reflective writing began via education research, with teachers and researchers wanting to know if there were evidence-based, replicable ways of getting students to learn. All the reflective cycles you come across are models based on education research. They are frameworks that have in some way been proven to challenge you and get you thinking about how to grow as a professional.

Two well-known reflective cycles are the Rolfe cycle and, as mentioned, the Gibbs Cycle (1998), the latter being the most well-known reflective cycle.

The Rolfe Cycle

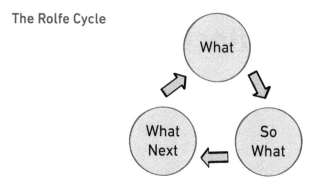

© Rolfe and Freshwater (2001) *Critical Reflection for Nursing and the Helping Professions:*
A User's Guide, Red Globe Press, used by permission of Bloomsbury Publishing plc

The Gibbs Cycle

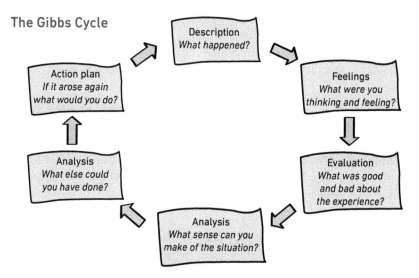

© Gibbs (1998) *Learning by Doing: A guide to teaching and learning methods.* Further
Education Unit. Oxford Polytechnic: Oxford.*

You can also look at the Kolb cycle; Bass is a midwifery-specific one;
and there are a few others you might come across (Bolton and
Delderfield 2018: 52–8). As midwifery lecturer Michelle Tant says:

It doesn't matter which reflective model you use as long as you can justify
your use of it and demonstrate how you used it effectively. Gibbs is a good,
simple one. Others, like John's model, or Kolb, can give you the opportunity
to go a bit deeper and so might be worth considering as you get into
second and third year. At the university I work at we provide an overview
of the various models and students can make their own judgement call on
which model works best for them, their assignment and the situation.

*This book is now available to download as an e-book from the website of the Oxford Centre
for Staff and Learning Development, Oxford Brookes University at http://www.brookes.
ac.uk/ocsld/publications/

If you're just starting out you might want to use the Gibbs Cycle, as it has six stages to follow and clear questions to answer. If you have a reason for using a cycle, mentioning this can help you gain marks.

Why we resist reflections

Reflections are an exercise in uncertainty. Midwifery situations are often too complicated to have a single best solution. In addition, examining our actions can quickly become personal, as looking after women and pregnant people in challenging situations is always going to require some management of our emotions. There are invisible circumstances and subconscious elements at play. As a student midwife, you will likely be busy and the last thing you will want to do some days is slow down and consider how all of these factors are contributing to care. But if you're a counsellor you are expected to have your own therapy sessions so you have some support around your reactions. Reflections are useful for similar reasons.

Reflections also cover the 'put your own oxygen mask on first' concept. It's easier to advocate for clients if you have self-awareness of your feelings and needs. If you add some consideration of policies and guidelines, and include some critique of relevant literature, you have a lot of tools at your disposal. In short, writing reflections can feel emotionally exposing and be hard work in terms of reading around the subject. But hopefully, you can see how useful they are.

Example reflective assignment [1]

Let's consider how you might approach a reflective assignment task.

The brief is:

> Reflect on a situation in practice in which a midwifery client experienced a threat to the health of their baby. Use the Gibbs Reflective Cycle. [3,000 words, +/- 10%]

This is a longer reflective assignment because I wanted to choose something we can get our teeth into, but this means I have included only relevant sections of it. For a complete but shorter reflection, see Example 2.

Planning your reflection

Broadly speaking you can use the same process as you would for any other essay while using a reflective cycle to guide you (if you're finding planning confusing, Chapter Two will break things down into more detail and might be worth revisiting).

> **Assess Question > Read Relevant Literature > Critique Care Given > Critique Literature > Structure Outline Using a Reflective Cycle > Write**

Remember that the stages are not discrete; you'll move back and forth as needed. Many students start by writing an account of what happened and work through the stages of the cycle sequentially. I like to start by looking at the evidence, at least briefly, so I can start to think about what kind of conclusion I'm building towards. I find this helps me focus on the research that is most applicable.

To give you an idea of how much detail to go into, have a look at how I would allocate word count.

Now let's take a closer look at the elements of a reflection that do not feature in a typical essay assignment.

Box 5.1: Approximate word count outline for a reflective assignment, 3,000 words, using the Gibbs Reflective Cycle

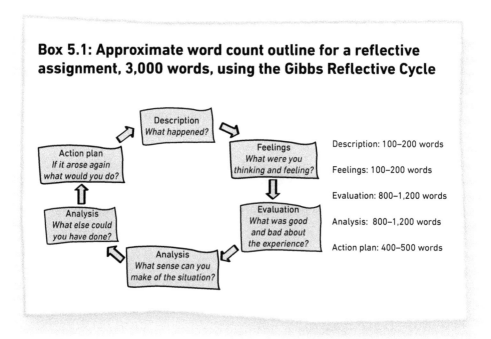

The Description and Feelings Sections

In the description and feelings sections of your reflection, you will be documenting an inner experience. However, this doesn't mean writing informally; you should be as factual as possible, and you need to be unambiguous, which means writing without idioms (to be clear, the whole of a reflection should be written in first person, it just needs to be formal in tone).

Table 5.1: Writing style guide for reflections

Less academic way of phrasing description and feelings sections	More academic way of writing description and feelings sections
So I needed to go back to the drawing board ...	The reassurance and information I provided was helpful, but not comprehensive enough to support the client, meaning I needed to ask a qualified professional to step in. This was disappointing ...
I was ecstatic when my care was praised ...	Both my practice supervisor and the client gave me positive feedback as the information I offered was clear, relevant and evidence-based. This helped increase my confidence ...
I was pretty sure it was going well ...	Once I gained experience and knew the trust guidelines on monitoring fetal growth, I began to feel more comfortable with this skill.
My stomach dropped.	I became aware of the distress of the client, and became concerned that I had not provided adequate information and support at the last appointment. My emotions were disappointment and shame.

If you have trouble writing about your emotions, know that many of us find this hard. Some researchers suggest adults can generally only identify three emotions as they are feeling them: happy, sad and angry (Brown 2021: xxi). However, there are many nuances, and though there is no consensus about how to classify human emotions, a good place to start is the sociologist Brené Brown's 'Eighty-Seven Emotions and Experiences' table, which can be found online (2022).

It can feel jarring to bring your inner world out in an assignment. You only need to reveal what feels right to you, but if you can identify your feelings, neurobiology research suggests that this will help you process them, allowing you to learn from the situation and take further action (Brown 2021: 279). If you can show these steps in your reflection, it will help you get higher marks.

In this example reflection, the task was to examine a clinical situation in which a client experienced a threat to the health of their baby. I can think of many situations which would be suitable. The following is an example I've adapted from one of my own reflections, and I've written it from the point of view of a student midwife.

Box 5.2: Description section for example reflective assignment [1]

I initially met Fatimah at her booking appointment when she was 8 weeks pregnant with her second baby. She had enjoyed a straightforward pregnancy and normal birth with her first. The next time I saw her, she was 28+6/40 and at her first obstetric appointment, which consisted of a scan and a discussion with the consultant about the diagnosis of Small for Gestational Age (SGA) fetus. She appeared to be calm, pleased with care, and able to ask questions. I also attended Fatimah's next community midwife appointment, which ended in Fatimah discussing her concerns about early IOL (Induction of Labour) or possible caesarean birth. She was able to discuss her fears with my practice supervisor, who is her named midwife. Fatimah was crying and stated she was upset because she felt her baby was at risk and she didn't understand what was happening.

Box 5.3: Feelings section for example reflective assignment [1]

On the day of Fatimah's obstetric appointment, I was nervous to be working in the Fetal Medicine Clinic. I had been told to sit in during an obstetric consultant appointment to gain experience of complex care. I was apprehensive about my level of knowledge in comparison to the obstetrician. I was pleased when Fatimah was the patient attending the appointment, as she was known to me from community care. She recognized me and I was proud to be a memorable student and happy to provide some continuity. I was concerned when the obstetrician talked about SGA but pleased when Fatimah seemed to understand. When I was working with my practice supervisor back at our community clinic, and saw Fatimah was our next client, I felt confident because I felt I could provide useful information and offer continuity of care. This made me happy, because as a student I often feel unsure about my role and fearful about taking up too much time when I need teaching or support. When Fatimah was upset, I felt disappointed that I had not provided the information or support she needed in the obstetric appointment, and ashamed as my practice supervisor was able to provide ideas and emotional support that seemed helpful for Fatimah, whereas I could not.

The evaluation and analysis section

The next prompts from the Gibbs Reflective Cycle are evaluation and analysis of events. 'Evaluation' and 'analysis' are concepts you would use in other assignments, so you may want to look at Chapter Two again for further help. In brief, think about the question you're trying to answer. In this example it would be: How best can midwives improve care for clients experiencing a diagnosis of SGA?

The Gibbs Reflective Cycle is often presented in study guides with prompt questions like 'what sense can I make of the situation?' and 'What knowledge – my own or others (for example academic literature) – can help me understand?' Writing out answers to these questions can help you fill the evaluation and analysis section of reflections with learning that will be easily recognized by tutors and their mark schemes.

Resources could include:

- hospital or trust policies
- national or international guidelines
- guidance from relevant midwifery or obstetric professional organizations
- research on which the guidelines or policies are based
- qualitative research that looks at the experiences of clients
- professional blogs and articles about similar issues which you could use to compare and contrast with your experience.

Depending on the length of your reflection, and how detailed it needs to be, you might also want to look at a research guide to help you critique studies and/or a textbook to help you think about anatomy and physiology.

Make notes as you read, and be sure to include references so when you come to write this section you can build your reference list. You can then choose the points you want to write about and add these to the outline of your reflection.

The action plan section

Your action plan should show how you would improve things next time. Ideally, your reflection will contain a chain of reasoning flowing from your original experience, through to evaluation and analysis, and to what you learned. My action plan here is also the conclusion for this assignment.

Box 5.4: action plan and conclusion sections for reflective assignment [1]

The decisions Fatimah needs to make are complex and the literature identifies concerns around clients feeling like they need to make decisions in line with their caregivers' opinions (Kirkup 2015; Ockenden 2022). The *Montgomery v Lanarkshire Health Board* case (2015) shows that informed choice can be neglected and relying only on expert opinion without offering informed choice is not a legally or ethically correct path. As a student only a few months into my second year of training, I do not yet have the level of information I would like to be able to support clients like Fatimah during complex obstetric conversations.

However, in order to support Fatimah, I could have used my own feelings of apprehension to remind me to ask the obstetrician questions. If a subject is new to us, we may be in some ways identifying with the experience of the client (Brown 2018), as they are also new to the situation. As a student midwife, empathy may be more easily achieved as my perspective is not yet from a place of 'freeze', as described in Lewin's learning model. It is also typical and positive for me to be feeling uncertain, and concerned, as these feelings are consistent with realizing I do not know something and are a step towards gaining skills and knowledge around advocacy (David 2013).

Though I was unhappy that I couldn't support Fatimah better during the obstetric appointment, I will take this as a learning experience. It would have been appropriate to ask Fatimah if she understood and if she had any further questions for the obstetric team during the appointment, and this may have identified some of her concerns and prompted more discussion (Birth Rights 2018; AIMS 2021). If I had known her feelings, I also might have been able to arrange a faster community appointment with Fatimah's named midwife. Another option would be an appointment with a consultant midwife who is available in our trust for clients wanting to make decisions outside the guidelines.

The existence of the Birth Rights charity, the *Montgomery v Lanarkshire Health Board* case (2015) and the other resources I have discussed in this reflection suggest to me that it is common to find advocacy in these kinds of situations to be challenging. However, I am feeling calmer that I have identified how I need to grow to work towards providing this support for clients when I qualify. A midwife's role in the promotion of normality and each client's trust in their own capabilities is identified by *The Lancet* midwifery series (2014). I feel this role is one of the weightiest and most complicated aspects of midwifery practice.

I hope to learn more about supporting clients with complex medical needs, using my academic assignments and placements to help me gain experience and knowledge. I also plan to attend a conference in February of this year that focuses on how to support normality in childbearing. This will be a good opportunity for me to ask questions, especially as some sessions are led by obstetricians and other members of the multidisciplinary team.

Confidential information and other challenges

Before we move on to the next example reflection, it's worth considering how you will uphold the confidentiality of the clients you are writing about. To do this, ensure you don't mention the trust you're working at or any other identifying features. In addition, if you're writing about a piece of care that you know didn't go that well, or had a poor outcome, make sure you send your tutor a copy of the draft you're working on so they can advise you on how to handle it. Sometimes students have found writing about a mistake they made or an issue that came up has many ramifications (NHS 2017). There may be incident forms to put in and processes to follow that should be prioritized before a graded reflection should take place.

Box 5.5: Top tips for achieving high marks

1. Just like with essay assignments, in-depth critical analysis will help you get high marks. Anything you say that's at all contestable should have a reference with some evidence backing it up.

2. Further your discussion by finding academic or other worthy sources that either agree or disagree with you, and compare and contrast with your own experience.

3. When midwives are practising they tend to hold the power in the relationship because clients don't have a professional level of experience or expertise (Murphy-Lawless 2018). Reflections are a good place to explore the culture of midwifery, what this power dynamic means for ourselves and clients, and how best to work in true partnership with clients.

4. It's easy for the best of us to go off on a tangent. If you have not made a detailed plan and are instead working through the reflective cycle stages one by one, keep the assignment brief and cycle to hand and tick off parts as you write them.

5. It might be helpful to know that the Bass Model of Holistic Reflection was designed based on midwifery philosophy and values. Though it might be a little too complex for the first reflection you write, it could be a very impressive cycle to use as you progress through your course. Perhaps check with your tutors about using it (Sweet et al. 2019).

Example of a reflective assignment [2]

The following is a reflection from a first-year student midwife undertaking an early placement. It uses the Rolfe reflective model (2001) with its 'What? So What? Now What?' questions, which offers a simple and efficient way of demonstrating learning.

This reflection would also be suitable for inclusion in a portfolio. Sometimes the reflections you keep in a portfolio are graded, but sometimes they are required but not graded, as they are more about prompting you to build the habit of writing reflections. You can decide how much time and energy to give each reflection depending on this factor.

Box 5.6: Reflection on taking venous blood for the first time – 02/02/22

Names and other identifying features have been changed to ensure confidentiality (Nursing and Midwifery Council (NMC), 2018)

Using the reflective model from Rolfe et al. (2001)

What:

This reflection is about taking booking bloods from a grand multiparous woman called April. April was 8+1/40 based on her Last Menstrual Period (LMP), and so was being offered antenatal screening as detailed in The National Institute for Health and Care Excellence (NICE) Antenatal care guidelines (2021).

My practice supervisor and I had called at April's house to conduct her booking in appointment. This home visit was at April's request as she had experienced 5+ previous miscarriages and felt it was unfair to let her other children know she was pregnant again as the chance of further miscarriage was high. Therefore the appointment had to be convenient for her so she could arrange childcare for her youngest children, and to ensure her older children were at school. This care was appropriate based on the recommendation in Better Births that maternity caregivers provide community care tailored to the needs of clients (NHS England 2016).

My practice supervisor offered April verbal and written information on the screening process, and April said she understood and that her stance on screening had not changed since her previous pregnancy, and wanted to proceed.

This was my initial attempt at venepuncture as a student midwife. After asking April if I could take blood, and explaining to her I was a student and just starting to learn this skill, April stated she was happy for me to go ahead. My practice supervisor then reminded me of the elements of the procedure; getting the sharps bin ready, having an alcohol wipe ready, having cotton wool for pressure afterwards ready, bottles having been labelled and needle ready. I also had washed my hands thoroughly, and before I started assembling equipment, I used alcohol gel. My practice supervisor talked me through my actions as I applied the tourniquet, visualized the median cubital vein which was bouncy and easily palpated, and entered it with the needle (Edwards 2021: 70). Taking blood went smoothly and there were no concerns. I used a safety needle with a needle cover, which the World Health Organisation (WHO) identifies as key for the protection of community-based healthcare workers (WHO 2010).

So what:

Before the procedure started, I felt nervous and apprehensive of causing April any pain. During the procedure I made an effort to be calm, concentrating on following my practice supervisor's instructions. After the procedure I felt elated as it had gone well; April told me she had felt very little pain.

The procedure was effective in taking 5 bottles of blood needed to test for Full Blood Count (FBC) (otherwise known as 'Hb' or 'iron count'), blood group and rhesus D status, sickle cell anaemia and thalassaemia, rubella, HIV and syphilis, Hepatitis B, and any antibodies in the blood which could cause harm to the fetus. All of these tests needed to be carried out so extra care or treatment could be given if necessary and essential information be assimilated for the wellbeing of the mother and the fetus. I was able to perform the procedure effectively because my practice supervisor gave me information as I was performing the actions, and she had a lot of clinical experience. The vein chosen was not thin enough to collapse, the vein was entered at a 30-degree angle to prevent collapse and the vacutainers were pulled backwards slowly and steadily to prevent the needle from moving (WHO 2010).

What next:

An area I would like to develop is my knowledge of antenatal screening as I didn't feel able to offer information to April. I know that clients can feel pressured to make decisions in line with their caregivers' wishes, (NHS England 2016) and I had little input into April's ability to make an informed choice. However, this reflection is focused on the clinical skill of venepuncture so I will aim to write a reflection that addresses antenatal screening in more detail in another reflection.

I have learned a lot about the procedure of taking venous blood, for instance, using the tourniquet, asking the patient to squeeze their fist to make the vein more visible, entering with the needle at a 30-degree angle and so on (WHO 2021; Edwards 2021: 70). I have also developed confidence in my ability to do the procedure while supervised. Next time I would like to take an even more active role, for instance finding the vein on my own, although still checking with my practice supervisor.

Though I handwrote the vacutainers on this occasion due to a printer not being available, in our community midwifery team, it is normal to use point of care stickers printed just before or after sampling. These show name, NHS number, surname, date of birth, and the date and time of the procedure. These stickers have been shown to reduce errors in labelling blood due to, for instance, misspelling of a client's name (WHO 2010). This is an important consideration as having to repeat taking a blood sample would be frustrating for both April and the team looking after her, would cause April unnecessary extra pain, and in the worst-case scenario, lead to an error in care such as mislabelling leading to a 'never event' of an ABO-incompatible transfusion.

Next time I would want to practise using stickers, however, I was pleased to practise handwriting the vacutainers as it is a necessary skill, as proved in this case. My practice supervisor also told me that knowing how to handwrite a blood group sample can be important during obstetric emergencies. If a printer is not to hand, accurately handwriting a sample can ensure a recent blood group result is available so that the correct type of blood transfusion can be made ready. Although rhesus negative blood that is suitable for any patient of any blood type is always available in our tertiary unit, this is a finite resource and the best practice would be to have a correct blood type ready for transfusion (Royal College of Obstetricians and Gynaecologists (RCOG) 2016).

I look forward to being able to reliably take blood autonomously and label it even in fast-paced emergency situations, and will continue to look for opportunities to practise this skill, with supervision, and where midwifery clients are happy for students to undertake venepuncture on them.

References:

Nursing and Midwifery Council (NMC) (2018). *The Code Professional standards of practice and behaviour for nurses and midwives Nursing and Midwifery Council.* Nmc.org.uk [Online]

National Institute for Health and Care Excellence (NICE) (2021). *Overview | Antenatal care | Guidance | NICE.* nice.org.uk. [Online]

NHS England (2016). *Better Births: Improving outcomes of maternity services in England – A Five Year Forward View for maternity care.* England.nhs.uk. [Online]

Edwards, A. (2020). *Antenatal midwifery skills: survival guide.* London: Routledge. P.70

World Health Organisation (WHO) (2010). *Guideline on drawing blood: best practices in phlebotomy.* euro.who.int [Online]

Royal College of Obstetricians and Gynaecologists (RCOG) (2016). *Prevention and Management of Postpartum Haemorrhage (Green-top Guideline No. 52).* Rcog.org.uk. [Online]

To conclude

If I were in charge of organizing maternity care and had an unlimited budget, I might implement free counselling support for students and qualified midwives. This would look something like an hour a week of relaxed but focused conversation about practice with an experienced midwife who's also a psychotherapist. But that's currently an unrealistic thing to provide, and, besides, there are advantages to you being able to assess your practice independently. The more reflections you write, the more you're more likely to be practising in a thoughtful, evidence-based way.

It's worth mentioning that though you will need to write formal reflections for your course and to maintain registration as a qualified midwife, writing informal reflections can also be helpful. I have a fancy pen some friends bought me for my 30th birthday and a few A4 blank notebooks with cool covers that I use for freehand writing about anything that's upsetting me in practice. I don't include the real names of clients and to be honest, I doubt anyone else could read my handwriting, but I do find capturing my thoughts to be soothing. It's also fascinating to look back on events that I've half-forgotten about, and it's easier to unpack things when some time has gone by. To find out more about my process, have a look at the midwifediaries.com blog post 'Midwifery Reflections and My Personal Strategy'.

6 Engaging with Research

Introduction

When learning about research as a student midwife, you're likely to come across the word 'appraisal'. To paraphrase Dr Sara Wickham, all appraisal means is working out what value to put on the particular piece of research you're looking at (2006: 1). As an undergraduate, you will likely do this by trying to understand the type of research, working out why it was done and identifying how it is different from other studies that have gone before it. This is a challenging task for a few reasons. Firstly, research papers are densely written due to journal word count limits, so you usually have to read them a few times to unpack what's going on. In addition, you'll need to work out where a piece of research fits into current evidence, so there's often reading you need to do alongside the research paper itself. You'll also need maths skills, as results are calculated using statistical tests, and presented via tables and graphs.

What I'm hoping to offer in this chapter is peer support. I will be signposting to experts in the field, whose work can offer a lot more guidance than I can. But I know that when learning something new it helps to hear how someone else has tackled challenges. I have to break things down and my basic strategy comes down to reading the research and making a list of hard questions as I go. I then try to answer these questions using common sense, research guides, resources like Khan Academy and YouTube, and occasional help from lectures, academic advisers at the library, or specialist midwives. I find research appraisal really difficult but it's also very rewarding.

Research guides

These are the books that I continually refer back to:

- Dr Sara Wickham's *Appraising Research into Childbirth* (2006)
- Dr Trisha Greenhalgh's *How to Read a Paper* (2019)
- Dr Amy Brown's *Informed is Best* (2019)

These have been most useful to me as e-books, as being able to jump around the text to the relevant areas and do keyword searches is what I need when trying to understand what's going on in a piece of research. But I do like physical books, and having Sara Wickham's workbook as a hard copy made it easier to work with, as I could look at the double page spreads.

Getting started

Broadly speaking, quantitative research is about numbers, and qualitative is about words and feelings. As a starting point, there is a short story called 'Cerridwyn and the Pixies: A Holiday Fairytale' that you might want to read. This draws attention to how different types of research are suited to finding different types of information. You can find it on Dr Sara Wickham's website or in her *Appraising Research into Childbirth book* (2006: 160)

If you're just beginning to read research, the following quick tips might be helpful.

- If you can afford it, invest in two computer monitors, or else use 'split-screen' to bring up two copies of the study side by side. This means you can read the text and look at any charts or graphs simultaneously without scrolling around and losing your place. Split-screen also helps if you're wanting to check or follow references at the same time as reading the text.

- Otherwise, consider printing the research and handwriting questions and comments in the margins. Ask yourself 'What don't I understand?' The questions you identify might feel unfocused when you're writing them but when you re-read them you'll pick up on important patterns or themes.

- Take breaks. If you find a study confusing, a lot of the time it's because you're missing a key concept, or you're trying to use a lot of new ideas at once. If you don't understand straight away, come back to it. I'll give a study maximum of three reads to see what I can get out of it and then give myself a break of a day or so. After some breathing space things often click into place.

- Don't forget how useful CTRL+F (on Windows) or Command+F (on Mac) are to search for a particular word, rather than scrolling through the document you're working with.

- The research guides above will give you checklists of questions to work through. This can be useful – or overwhelming. Try and think about what the most important questions are in the context of the study. If your university has suggested a checklist, perhaps ask a lecturer what the most important questions are and what you should spend most time and attention on.

- A lot of what you will be doing as you start looking at research is getting used to the ideas and technical language.

- Once you get going, you'll probably find lots of things to comment on that question the validity of the research you're appraising. However, know that research doesn't have to be perfect to be useful and researchers never get it 100 per cent right as the odds are so stacked against them. Though you should be identifying ways in which the research could be unreliable, working out why certain compromises have been made and understanding why the researchers have made certain choices is often more helpful than disregarding the research altogether.

How research is presented

Most research starts with an abstract, and is then set out as IMRAD, i.e. Introduction, Methods, Results, and Discussion. Use the books mentioned above to read about these components, which will give you points to think about or comment on in an assignment.

Types of research

If we're thinking about the basic differences between research, broadly speaking, there are two kinds: experimental and observational. Experimental studies mean a researcher has set up the study by providing an intervention. Observational studies mean researchers observe an intervention or phenomenon that already exists. Experimental research is often thought of as a more powerful kind of research, especially if you have a control group and properly randomize which participant goes into each group (Rees 2011). You can also get mixed methods studies which combine the two.

Here is a basic, simple diagram of different kinds of research and the 'hierarchy' of evidence.

The Hierarchy of Research Evidence

Strongest Evidence *

Systematic reviews of randomized controlled trials

Randomized controlled trials

Non-randomized trials, case-controlled studies, observational studies

Qualitative research

Expert opinion from panels or committees

Expert opinion

Weakest Evidence *

*Assuming trials are all well designed

(Aldcroft 2018; Brown 2019; Greenhalgh 2019; Wickham 2006)

However, boundaries between different kinds of research are more fluid than the diagram above suggests, and studies can have overlapping factors. Also, the hierarchy of evidence is more complicated than 'systematic reviews of randomized controlled trials (RCTs) are the best'. For a start, the research hierarchy doesn't take into account the feasibility of each type of study as, for instance, it is unethical to randomly assign people to a caesarean birth so you can do a randomized controlled trial on them. It would also be impossible to blind participants and researchers to the different groups as a caesarean is a very noticeable bit of surgery. Later on in this chapter, I'll explain what a case series is, but, for now, know that based on the hierarchy of evidence, it's a type of study with low significance. But in some situations, especially when you need to put a study together quickly to alert professionals to something dangerous, it can be a perfect choice. In addition to this, qualitative research, which is fairly low down in the table, can get to information that quantitative research can't touch. And not just in terms of understanding emotional well-being; it's saved lives on many occasions.

As well as 'systematic review', you'll also see the term 'meta-analysis' which means bringing together evidence from different pieces of research and using maths to come to more informed conclusions. To quote Amy Brown 'every study has limitations, but if you bring all the data together it will help reduce them'. The power also comes from the increased number of individuals being studied, as, in general, the bigger the sample size, the more informed the results (Brown 2019: 1136).

You can also get systematic reviews of studies that are not RCTs, but are still useful. My favourite example of a systematic review is represented in the Cochrane Library logo. It's a forest plot from different studies looking at whether an injection of corticosteroids given to women or birthing people in premature labour can help improve survival and outcomes. Before the systematic review corticosteroids were not given in these circumstances uniformly, it depended on where you were in the country. The forest plot was brilliant because it showed clear evidence that 'corticosteroids given to women who are about to give birth prematurely can save the life of the newborn child'. This evidence had been amassed since the 1960s but it took until 1992 for the Royal College of Obstetricians and Gynaecologists to issue a guideline on the subject which every hospital took note of. Before this, babies needlessly suffered and died. My brother was born prematurely in 1994, so every time I see the Cochrane symbol I feel grateful and a little in awe of how powerful research can be (Cochrane Collaboration 2017).

But on the other hand, not all systematic reviews are done well. If the studies that are brought together are poorly designed, or the maths has been done badly, you'll just end up with compounded mistakes.

Quantitative research

Types of quantitative research

Randomized controlled trials

As just discussed, RCTs are traditionally thought of as the gold standard of research evidence. This is because they eliminate bias in a structured way. RCT participants are assigned in advance to different interventions, using random allocation. RCTs work best when you have a simple question to answer, like 'Does this drug work or not?' If you've got any kind of human behaviour involved, it can become hard to keep your groups randomized.

A good point that illustrates this is related to the following choice. Hopefully, everyone in an RCT does exactly what they're told. But in reality, researchers usually have to decide how to analyse their data using one of the following mutually exclusive strategies.

1. Per protocol: the researchers only include compliant participants. The issue with this is that they now have a group that's been shaped by that choice. You get inherent self-selected differences. How can the researchers be sure of what they're interpreting?

2. Intention to treat: the researchers include every participant, regardless of whether they stuck with the treatment assigned or not. This might provide insight that's closer to what happens in the real world, but the issue is you end up with groups who haven't done exactly what you suggested when you set things up. So how can you be sure of what you're analysing? (Brown 2019: 189)

As well as RCTs, you also get 'Other Controlled Trials' where randomization isn't possible. In 'How to Read a Paper' Trisha Greenhalgh writes about a cluster trial from the early twentieth century that allocated patients in a hospital to different diets. One ward full of patients was fed meals with white rice and another ward was served brown. Their eventual symptom or easing of symptoms suggested that the disease was linked to diet deficiency, in this case, thiamin deficiency, otherwise known as Beri Beri disease. This is an example of a controlled trial without randomization (Greenhalgh 2019: 39). Randomization would have been so hard to achieve – you'd need a hospital catering system that managed to get a specific random diet to each patient on a ward, for a month or so, in a reliable and trackable way, and to be successful in preventing those patients from ever swapping their meal with someone else. It is obviously far easier to just assign ward A to one diet and ward B to another. It's important to know that sometimes achieving true randomization is impractical, but actually there are times when it doesn't matter much, and the result you get will be useful anyway.

Cohort studies

Cohort studies are a type of longitudinal study, which means that they follow a group of people through time. Researchers repeat measurements at specified intervals, and groups that differ based on their exposure to a factor are compared. One famous cohort study followed 40,000 male British doctors and showed a link between smoking and mortality. These days cohort studies can use digital patient records to include several thousand participants at once, making them very powerful (Greenhalgh 2019: 37–9).

Case-control studies

These studies look at participants with a disease and compare them to similar participants who don't have the disease, i.e. a 'case' and a matched 'control' group. The key is that the control group are chosen to be as similar as possible to the case group. Again, patient records access has made it a lot easier to conduct these. Case-control studies are important for looking at rare diseases or outcomes. However, they are less reliable than cohort studies in proving a connection between factors and instead show only an association. Sudden Infant Death Syndrome (SIDS) is often studied using case-control research (Brown 2019: 132; Greenhalgh 2019: 40).

Cross-sectional studies

These are sometimes called 'cross-sectional survey' studies. They're like a snapshot in time. Because of this, they can't prove causation. But these can be useful for identifying areas that need more in-depth study or for following up on whether a screening test was useful or not (Brown 2019: 132–4; Greenhalgh 2019: 40–1).

Qualitative research

If I ever get to do research, I hope it will be qualitative. Qualitative research guides give instructions on how to find data that is 'rich' and 'thick' and suggest researchers aim to write their findings up so readers 'almost feel they are there' with the participants. All of these are ways of describing how qualitative research helps us to better understand human beings and their experience of the world (Rees 2011: 70). Qualitative researchers get their data from observation, interviews, focus groups and sometimes online social media or written sources like newspapers.

You will also find the word 'inductive' to describe qualitative research, which means you start with an observation and work towards a theory. This is as opposed to 'deductive' reasoning, which is concerned with testing a hypothesis and so applies to quantitative research (Wickham 2006: 154).

Types of qualitative research

Ethnography

This is a branch of anthropology. Researchers try to understand a particular culture, sometimes through participation and sometimes through observation (described as participatory and non-participatory methods) (Brown 2019: 127; Bryman 2012: 464–7).

Phenomenology

This comes from the word phenomenon and is to do with understanding first-person experiences using interviews, written materials or group discussion (Brown 2019: 127–8).

Grounded theory

Like phenomenology, but you compare all your data until you have an emerging theory (Brown 2019: ch. 8). All your interviews with participants have to confirm your theory. If you find a human experience that doesn't match your theory, you have to throw your theory out and start again. I was intrigued to note that one researcher says that grounded theory is 'virtually impossible' to fully understand without conducting it (Brown 2013: 251).

Questioning the validity of qualitative research

You could argue that qualitative research is not very reliable because it's essentially an exercise in stacking quotes together, and you can therefore make it show whatever you want (Stewart 2010: 77–8). But there is plenty that researchers can do to make sure their findings are trustworthy. For example, they can:

- gain ethical approval so the methodology will have undergone some scrutiny;

- keep a reflective diary to self-evaluate and to share their methods with other researchers;
- use a variety of different participants;
- use multiple methods;
- declare particular biases or interests so the findings can be interpreted with this in mind (qualitative research comes with the understanding that all researchers will have a particular point of view that can't be unpicked from the findings, but researchers declare this and work with it as they go);
- take the research findings back to the participants and see whether they agree or disagree.

(Rees 2011: ch. 4; Stewart 2010: 77–8)

Quantitative research can find information that qualitative research methods would find very hard to capture. I can adapt my practice according to quantitative research outcomes but how clients feel about their care is not something that's easily assessed with numbers. In her *Gathering in the Knowledge* online course (2021) Sara Wickham discussed a piece of research on birth trauma:

Cos it's not acceptable to say – 'I can't stand my baby' is it?

(Molloy et al. 2021)

See what 'rich, thick' description means?

And Amy Brown cites some research undertaken in places like Liberia and Sierra Leone during the Ebola crisis. Qualitative researchers were trusted because they'd been part of the community, and they had real relationships to draw on. They were, therefore, able to identify that ritual washing of bodies was part of the problem, something that strict quantitative research wouldn't have found (Brown 2019: 134)

In terms of assessing appropriate sample sizes for qualitative research, look at the following:

Saturation occurs when adding more participants to the study does not result in additional perspectives or information. Glaser and Strauss (1967) recommend the concept of saturation for achieving an appropriate sample size in qualitative studies. Other guidelines have also been recommended. For an ethnography, Morse (1994) suggested approximately 30 – 50 participants. For grounded theory, Morse (1994) suggested 30 – 50 interviews, while Creswell (1998) suggested only 20 – 30. For phenomenological studies, Creswell (1998) recommends 5 – 25 and Morse (1994) suggests at least six. There are no specific rules when determining an appropriate sample size in qualitative research. Qualitative sample size may best be determined by the time allotted, resources available, and study objectives (Patton, 1990).

(Moran 2013)

Study types that can be both quantitative and qualitative

Case reports and case series

A case report is an article that describes and explains care given to an individual patient or client. Case reports are low down the research hierarchy because the evidence is drawn from a single person. But actually, clinicians do a lot of teaching via telling stories, which to my mind is pretty much a case report. It was a case report which identified phocomelia (absent limbs) in babies whose mothers had taken thalidomide, a morning-sickness drug. It's a good kind of research if you need to get the word out quickly (Greenhalgh 2019: 42).

For a midwifery example of a case report, you might want to read 'Lethal fetal anomalies: a case of bilateral renal agenesis' (Howes and Muscat 2015). This is an account of care given by independent midwife Virginia Howes as she looked after her client Natalie Lennard. Natalie laboured and gave birth to her son at home, despite the certain outcome of him not surviving. This is a good example of a case report as it helps expand our ideas about the choices clients can make in bereavement situations.

In a case series, case reports are grouped together. The number of case reports included should be big enough to find a significant result. Statistics are needed to work out exactly how big the sample size should be, depending on the level of certainty you're aiming for (Brown 2019: 225–6).

Case reports and case series can be thought of as qualitative or quantitative, or involve both types of methods, depending on content. It's worth pointing out that many types of studies can be combined, so you may come across qualitative research that has quantitative aspects, or vice versa.

Components of research

It's good to consider the kind of tools that researchers use to generate their data. The following are some common ones along with their advantages and disadvantages.

Questionnaires/surveys

Surveys can provide a fast and economical way of generating data, and are used in many different kinds of studies. They're useful as you can get really big sample sizes, they can be anonymous and are often straightforward to analyse.

However, the reliability of survey answers can be questionable, as they can be tedious to fill out. Also, they can mean people who don't speak English don't get a voice, and they perhaps won't capture more complex responses (Wickham 2006: 58). In addition, if it's a survey that is asking about something in the past, the responses might not be well remembered (Anderson 2010: 45)

How interested participants are in filling out surveys is a useful consideration too. Anything less than a 50 per cent response rate means the data isn't likely to be truly representative; the *British Medical Journal* usually doesn't take research based on surveys that have less than a 70 per cent response rate (Greenhalgh 2019: 186).

Ethical approval

It's not illegal to conduct human subject research without the approval of an ethics committee but it's very difficult to get funding or to get publication without this. In the aftermath of the Second World War, the Nuremberg Code and Declaration of Helsinki were set up which form the basis of ethical research guidance. Amy Brown has a superb write-up of this which illustrates why ethical research is so important (2019: ch. 13, 197).

In terms of midwifery research, it's important to assess whether participants know their confidentiality will be upheld, as, especially during qualitative research, uncertainty around this may alter what they say. Participants (or their carers/guardians) should give informed consent to take part, and they should be aware there will be no adverse consequences should they withdraw (Brown 2019: 197–9)

Peer review

Peer review means a paper has been given to other researchers, and comments have been received about its validity and importance.

Journals organize this process in order to work out what they should publish. Amy Brown has a lot of useful comments on this subject and points out that peer review can be affected by the internal politics of certain fields and personalities of the experts within them (2019: 163). But broadly speaking, peer review is undertaken by most good journals.

You can also look at the 'Impact Factor' which is an index based on the number of times a journal has been cited in the last year. I use Web of Science, a website that you can access with university logins. But bear in mind impact factors are likely to be low for birth research as the topic area has a relatively low readership (Brown 2019: 162–4).

Influences on research

The following are some common factors that influence the reliability of research. They may help you identify points to consider in a paper you're looking at.

Human behaviour

When it comes to research done on people there's always something interesting to comment on in terms of human behaviour. Think about who could have limited the reliability of the study. Was the study supposed to be blind but the people administering the intervention were aware of what it was? Could they have communicated something about it to the participants? Did the participants take the pill/read the information/do the exercise or just lie to the researchers about it? Did the participants actually remember what they'd done and report it correctly? (Brown 2019: 120–1; Wickham 2006: ch. 6)

Who declined?

It can also be a great idea to look at the number of participants who declined to be part of the study you're reading. An example from a few years ago is the ARRIVE trial which was a huge induction of labour study done in 2018 (Grobman et al.). The set-up was 3,062 primigravid women being assigned to induction at 39 weeks and 3,044 assigned to expectant management, i.e. waiting for them to labour naturally.

The study found that the induction group had a slightly reduced chance of having a caesarean. But out of 22,500+ women who were asked to be in the trial, only 6,000ish agreed. This means loads of women said 'I don't want to risk being induced'. Women interested in induction self-selected to be in the trial, which may well have impacted the results (do people keen on induction of labour progress better during an induction of labour? What do we know about oxytocin that suggests this could be the case?) (Brown 2019: 193).

Common confounding variables

A confounding variable is an extra variable which has not been taken into account. These can create false results. A classic example of a confounding variable is increased ice-cream consumption leads to more shark attacks. In fact, a more likely explanation is that an increase in temperature leads to increased ice-cream consumption, and also means more people go swimming in the sea, which leads to more shark attacks. So in this example, the weather is a confounding variable, as opposed to sharks somehow being affected by increased ice-cream sales.

In midwifery, there are a few common confounding variables. Think through the following:

- Consider whether the variables in the study came with any added extras. For instance, if a group of participants were given an intervention, did they get this dispensed by a healthcare professional who had an appointment with them? Perhaps it was the appointment rather than the pill that made them feel better?
- Was the dependent variable going to change over time anyway? For instance, perhaps it was the dressing that worked but maybe the young, fit, healthy participants were going to heal up anyway?
- Did socioeconomic, geographical or age factors influence the results?
- Was the study done at a particular time of year – did this have an impact on the activities, diet or free time of the participants?

(Brown 2019; Greenhalgh 2019; Wickham 2006)

Funding, conflict of interest and individual bias

Research helps us to systematically test hypotheses and prove or disprove ideas. However, the vast majority of medical research is done by 'rich white men who tend to do research they believe matters ... to other rich white men' (Brown 2019: 11).

We know that 27.4 per cent of undergraduates at UK universities are from Asian, Black, mixed or other backgrounds (Higher Education

Student Statistics 2021). But 'only 17% of UK academics are from Black and minority ethnic groups' (Higher Education Staff Statistics (HESA) 2021). Something is happening that means people from Black and minority ethnic groups are underrepresented at higher levels. Also 'a decent size trial can cost more than people's homes to conduct' (Brown 2019: 193). This means that the body of research we have is going to be more or less trustworthy depending on what kind of group we belong to, and whether that group has traditionally had that kind of money to spend on research. To get published you usually have to say where you got your funding from and to get funding you have to persuade a university or sometimes a drug company that your research is worth doing. You can see how we end up with an evidence base largely drawn from those in power. Researchers in developing world countries, for example, won't be able to do the kinds of research that we think are 'the best', which leaves gaping holes in our evidence base for people from particular places and cultures (Brown 2019: ch. 7).

Birth research is the best scientific evidence we have for midwifery but it's nowhere near able to predict what's going to happen to an individual client, especially if that client is Black, brown, doesn't speak English, is differently able, or is LGBTQ+ (especially transgender or non-binary). This is because we as a society are not very interested in these people when it comes to research funding.

Other areas of bias you can think about:

- Knowledge is a 'complex and uncertain beast' (Greenhalgh 2019: 237) and how we choose facts from research and put them into guidelines has had a lot of legitimate criticism.

- Looking at the global picture, it's studies from North America or Europe that are most likely to be published (Brown 2019: 137).

- Amy Brown has some terrifying discussions of how little conflict of interest is declared, especially when it comes to formula milk companies. There is at least one documented case of a formula company outright fabricating results (2019: 117).

Tables, graphs and charts

Sara Wickham has a good write-up on interpreting tables. She suggests if you are confused by a table, go back to the study text and read through the relevant paragraphs (2006: 142–3). This strategy has worked for me a few times. Remember that the researchers might be using shorthand; for instance, I was looking at a Cochrane review recently and didn't know what 'PY' meant (answer: 'Person Years'). In the end, I had to go back to the main text and read through it. As soon as I knew what the acronym meant, everything else made sense.

There's also a good chapter on analysing graphs in *An Introduction to Research for Midwives* (Rees 2011: 184). You could start by identifying the type of graph you have, e.g. bar chart, histogram, pie chart, etc. But more important than knowing the type is any meaning you can find. If you have a graph to interpret, start by working out what the x-axis and y-axis mean. I've come across a few trials where the axes are labelled with the concept but no scale, so you're just supposed to infer what's going on from the text. This isn't best practice by the authors but you can usually work out what they're showing by looking at the kinds of figures in the text; what would be a common-sense pattern being shown, based on the numbers, and the title of the graph?

Otherwise, with both tables and graphs, it comes back to making a list of questions and trying to answer them. Eventually, it'll click and if it doesn't, try emailing the library with a copy of your study and your question. They will either be able to help or point you towards places to find out more.

Statistics

Many of us find understanding statistical tests difficult, but it's reassuring that even Trisha Greenhalgh who wrote *How to Read a Paper* tends to 'go into panic mode at the sight of ratios, square root signs and half-remembered Greek letters' (2019: 124). All I can say is that I burst a blood vessel in my eye writing this bit of the chapter (I wish I was joking) but I feel a lot better about statistics now.

I suggest using the Khan Academy website, YouTube and doing extra Googling as you go. I can now mostly get to the heart of what a piece of research is about and offer some sensible suggestions about the findings. I hope my pointers are helpful.

Ways of calculating the average

Before we tackle statistics, it's good to review the basic ways in which we can measure the 'centre' of different sets of numerical data. The mean, median, mode and range are useful to understand the central tendencies of data. We use different kinds in different settings (Khan Academy 2016).

Table 6.1: Understanding the central tendencies of data

Definition	Pros and Cons
Mean: add all results up and divide by the number of results	The mean is often a good average to calculate but only if your data is symmetrical and has no outliers. If there are extremes of data, like a very big or very small value, this can push the mean in one direction or another
Median: the midpoint value, if you've lined all the data up in order	The median is less sensitive to outliers than the mean but it doesn't tell us much about the outer edges of the data
Mode: the most common value	The mode can be great in a 'x is the most common experience' kind of way but it doesn't let us see much beyond that
Range: the difference between the biggest and smallest numbers	The range is good for telling us about the spread between the highest and lowest values but not a lot else
Interquartile Range (IQR): the difference between the 75th and the 25th percentiles of the data	This measures the spread of the data without being unduly influenced by outliers

(For a more detailed overview, see Wickham 2006: 148)

I'm about to move on to some more complex ideas, but before that I would like to mention that I only have a basic understanding of statistics and in many cases, I just trust the mathematicians involved in the research to know what they're doing. Statisticians are just as guilty of using jargon as midwives; in the same way as we'll say 'SROM' (Spontaneous Rupture Of Membranes), statistics has its own internal language and you need experience to be able to navigate it.

I ask Google lots of fiddly questions and refresh my knowledge for pretty much every study I read. And if I don't understand I tend to let it go and move on. Think of the statisticians involved as members of the multidisciplinary team – you can check their work but not with the same level of experience that you have available for midwifery-specific knowledge.

Standard deviation

You can look at Khan Academy (2019) or a statistics book to understand what standard deviation is, but essentially it's a way of expressing variation from the average. You calculate it by finding the average squared distance to the mean and then finding the square root of this. Usually what you need to do when looking at research is to compare a higher standard deviation to a lower standard deviation and know what that might mean when comparing different sets of data.

Moving on to specific knowledge on statistics, the two big ideas that have been most helpful for me to grasp are p-values and confidence intervals.

Big scary statistical ideas and tests

These get complicated so please don't worry about feeling confused. I'd be amazed if you understood the first time you came across these ideas. It's very normal to need a few sessions to feel comfortable, but the good news is, if you keep at it, this is all achievable knowledge.

P-values

The name 'p-value' is from 'probability' – it's just shorthand for saying 'probability value'. In research, everyone is obsessed with validity and reliability, but all knowledge is contestable and there's never a way to be 100 per cent certain about anything. So the most sensible thing we can do is get all of that uncertainty into a pile and keep an eye on it. A p-value is a way of talking about the likelihood of getting a result that was a chance finding. The preferred way of expressing p-values is as a decimal, with 1 meaning the result has certainly occurred by chance, and 0 meaning it certainly didn't occur by chance.

Say we're 99 per cent certain about something. We're 1 per cent uncertain about it. If we express this as a decimal this would mean we have a 0.01 level of uncertainty about it. So $p = 0.01$.

In statistics, they take the concept of being 95 per cent certain about something to be a useful benchmark. So a 5 per cent level of uncertainty, which as a decimal is 0.05.

When you conduct research and use statistics, you often start with a null hypothesis. This means a hypothesis that says some intervention or other is ineffective or has no impact. For instance, say you're interested in whether kids who live in a home with a cat end up taller than kids who live in a home without a cat. Your null hypothesis would be: living in a home with a cat has no impact on height.

You would then take the answer offered by your study and run some numbers and come up with a p-value. If this p-value was *below* 0.05 you could reject your null hypothesis, i.e. .e. 'living in a home with a cat has no impact on height' = wrong. So 'living in a home with a cat has an impact on height' = right.

If the p-value was 0.05 or more, we couldn't reject the 'kids living in a home with a cat has no impact on height' statement. We'd have no statistically significant certainty about what the heck was going on with cats and kids' height.

Therefore when you're looking at data in a trial you will be presented with p-values.

What I try to remember is that if you have a p-value less than 0.05, that's statistically significant. If it's 0.000005 that's incredibly statistically significant. If you have a p-value of above 0.05, say 0.06, your finding is not statistically significant and may be because of chance. If it's something like 0.9 that's *very* likely to be because of chance (Greenhalgh 2019: 72; Wickham 2006: 156).

Confidence intervals

As mentioned above, even with the best trial, and clearest result, we can't know anything for sure, we can just get pretty close. Confidence intervals are a way of expressing that thought. I think of confidence intervals like taking your car to a garage and getting an estimate of when it'll be ready. The mechanics say it'll probably be ready between 3.00 pm and 5.00 pm. But the real time your car will be ready is unknown. It could be ready at 2.00 pm, 4.15 pm, 6.00 pm or even tomorrow. But it's most likely to be somewhere between 3.00 pm and 5.00 pm.

You will get a 'point estimate', represented by a dot on graphs, which tends to be in the middle of the confidence interval. The point estimate is usually the mean. So with our garage example, it would be something like, 'We believe your car will be ready at 4.00 pm. But it's unlikely to be earlier than 3.00 pm or later than 5.00 pm.'

Confidence intervals look like this.

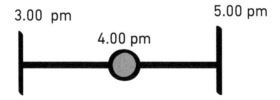

A confidence interval will often be expressed as a percentage. Researchers usually go for 95 per cent. This is arbitrary; people using statistics seem to like the 95 per cent thing; notice how it's the same amount as significance in p-values (0.05 = 5 per cent chance of it is not true, or 1/20 if you wanted it as a fraction).

You can do fancy maths equations depending on the type of data to get to your confidence interval of 95 per cent. Most people doing studies will use a specialist spreadsheet or online calculator to do this, or sometimes they will outsource to a statistician. A 95 per cent confidence interval means: 'there's a 95% chance that the interval that we get is good enough to contain the true value' (Massachusetts Institute of Technology 2014).

All you need to know to appraise research is that a confidence interval is a way of expressing a plausible margin of error. This is a complex concept, but there will be certain values that a confidence interval will not cross if you have a definitive (really reliable) result.

Say we're looking at a particular set of data where 1 is the line of null effect (i.e. the point where there is no difference between the intervention group and control group):

A confidence interval of (0.2, 0.6) doesn't cross 1 = definitive result.

A confidence interval of (0.75, 1.25) does cross 1 = not definitive result.

You will sometimes see them plotted on a graph like this:

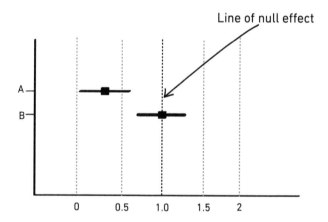

The point estimate (the squares on the graph) is quite often an average from the data, like a mean, but it can be other things too, you just have to figure it out as you read the paper.

You would be more trusting of a narrower estimate. So for example, if the garage said your car will be ready between 4.00 pm and 4.15 pm, that sounds much more promising than between 3.00 pm and 7.00 pm. In the same way, if you get a narrow interval in a study, you know this is more significant than a really big confidence interval (Greenhalgh 2019: 74; Wickham 2006: 157).

Other statistical tests

To start understanding statistical tests that are used in research, I recommend the YouTube video 'Statistics Made Easy' with Greg Martin (2019).

T-test

We'd use this test if we were comparing two groups (e.g. smokers vs non-smokers during pregnancy) and had continuous data (e.g. birthweight) and wanted to determine if the means of these two sets of data were different. We'd make a null hypothesis (smoking during pregnancy has no effect on birthweight). If the t-test showed a p-value of < 0.05, then we can reject the null hypothesis and conclude that there is a link between smoking and birth weight.

There are different kinds of t-tests that you can read about in statistics textbooks (Rees 2011: 176).

Chi-square test

This is pronounced 'kai', as in rhymes with pie. 'Chi' is a Greek letter, written as X.

If your data is categorical (e.g. hair colour: red, blonde, brown, black, other) and the variable you're predicting is also categorical (e.g. higher blood loss postnatally) then a chi-square test is suitable (Wickham 2006: 148).

ANOVA

This stands for Analysis of Variance. It's a similar idea to the t-test, in that it determines if there is a statistically significant difference between means of groups, where we have continuous data for those groups. However, the t-test is limited to two groups, whereas ANOVA can be used with any number. An example would be analysing whether dog weight is determined by the breed of the dog (Wickham 2006: 156).

Other Tests

Other tests that can come up in birth research include the F-test, Kruskal-Wallis test, Wilcoxon signed-rank test, Mann-Whitney U test and Z-test (Wickham 2006). My best advice is to look these up when you need them – your university library should be able to help you with a good textbook. If the research you're looking at appears to be on a fairly common topic but it features a test that's not in a basic statistics book, there's possibly some manipulation of the results going on (see Greenhalgh 2019: 68).

Odds ratios and risk ratios

An odds ratio is a measure of the relationship between exposure and an outcome. A risk ratio (also known as relative risk) is a measure of the risk of an event happening in one group compared with the risk in another group. There's a good explanation of this in *Informed is Best* (Brown 2019: 148) and a YouTube video on the subject made by Rahul Patwari (2015). To explain why we might need to know about these, let's consider cohort studies and case-control studies.

With a cohort study, you generally start with a group and follow it until some participants have experienced an outcome. From this, you can express the probability of something happening. This means you can find a risk ratio, which is a measure that can be applied to a whole population.

Where it would be too expensive or intrusive to do a cohort study, a case-control study can be used to estimate the prevalence of suspected factors in the general population. To do a case-control study, you start with participants who have experienced a certain outcome and then choose control participants who are similar but who did not experience that outcome. Since you don't start with a big group of people and follow them through, and instead, look at what happened in the past, the probability of something happening can't be given. Instead, you can give an odds ratio. You end up talking about the odds of a group having had something happen, in comparison to the control group who did not have that something happen.

An odds ratio is not as useful a measure as a risk ratio but it's still a pretty good statistic to have, and is sometimes the best way of considering an unusual condition or circumstance.

With both risk ratios and odds ratios, it's important to check the confidence intervals quoted by the study. If a confidence interval crosses 1, for instance, it is given as something like (0.99, 1.15); this means the findings are not statistically significant. If the confidence interval given doesn't cross 1, for instance (1.01, 1.28) then it is statistically significant (Greenhalgh 2019: 127).

When it comes to very rare occurrences or diseases, the risk ratio and odds ratio are pretty similar in terms of usefulness. They can both make small risks seem more significant than they are. Most of us need figures of absolute risk to grasp what's going on. To explain further, and taking an example from Amy Brown (2019: 154):

> An odds ratio might say that this particular course of action (y) means we are three times more likely to develop x.

The absolute risk might reveal that though this is true, we only had a 0.2 per cent risk of developing x in the first place, so if we do y we now have a 0.6 per cent risk of developing x, or a 99.4 per cent chance of not developing x.

When a tabloid says something like 'eating bananas means you are five times as likely to get cancer' they are usually deliberately creating alarming news using relative risk.

Correlation and regression

This is about looking at a study's variables and assessing their relationship. As one variable changes, the other may well also, and the strength of the relationship between the two things happening at the same time is known as correlation.

Correlation is often a weak standard of evidence and you can find correlations between things that are not at all related. Sara Wickham talks about a study that showed a relationship between higher stork population and increased homebirth (the researchers were mucking around, surely, but the data was for real) (2006: 152). Despite the issues, correlation can add to our existing body of knowledge about a topic and flag up a connection that needs further investigation. Using more complex models to analyse can help control for factors like age, income, ethnicity and so on.

Correlation is usually expressed as a correlation coefficient. This will be a number between -1 and 1. -1 means a negative correlation, and 1 means a positive correlation, and 0 means no correlation at all; the bigger the number in either direction, the bigger the correlation. This is referred to as an r value, or R value if it's for an entire population. See a great list of questions to ask when assessing whether researchers are right to use a correlation coefficient in *How to Read a Paper* (Greenhalgh 2019: 70).

Anything using the term 'regression' is about trying to look at how the variables interact and predicting what might come next. The *Brandon Foltz Statistics 101* (2020) videos on YouTube are great for understanding regression.

Linear regression is a way of looking for a relationship between variables. You can draw a line of best fit and then use it to make predictions. Multiple linear regression means you can look at multiple independent variables, like for instance blood pressure and blood sugar, and their impact on the dependent variable, on say, life span (Foltz 2020).

Logistic regression is used to find a probability of a binary outcome (with something like mortality, we're talking an outcome that's either yes or no, not continuous data like weight or height). I don't believe you have to understand the maths behind it, and researchers would use a computer to do this, as calculating logistic regression by hand would take years. Logistic regression was used in the birthplace study in the UK because the dependent variable was a binary outcome, i.e. i.e. neonatal mortality or morbidity, and the independent variable was where the birth took place (Brocklehurst et al. 2011).

And then you have multiple logistic regression which is the same thing as logistic regression but with more than two possible outcomes.

In terms of analysing the relationships between things, you get *univariate analysis* (which is straightforward, stuff like the mean, median and mode, and standard deviation, all to do with single variables), *bivariate analysis* which is to do with correlation and regression, which we covered above, and *multivariate analysis* which may also include regression, and I have to say sounds complicated, covers a lot of overlapping ground and is probably better off explained by someone better qualified than me (Wickham 2006: 152–3).

It's out of the scope of this book to go further into these ideas. Just take it question by question. As you know, I do a lot of Googling and flicking between my favourite e-books and YouTube videos.

Overall

- The best tip I've ever come across with research appraisal is to remember your conclusions have to be useful to the clients in your care. Try to imagine what this study means for your clients as individuals. Is there a group of people who have been missed out in this research – for instance, those with a particular medical condition? It may be that you have just healthy women/birthing people in your study, meaning this is a limitation for those who need medical input. Or the reverse may be true; perhaps this research doesn't apply to clients who have a physiological vaginal birth

- Your university should give you a research appraisal checklist, but if not you can find midwifery-specific ones in a textbook on midwifery research, for instance *An Introduction to Research for Midwives* by Colin Rees (2011).

- You could also see if your hospital has a journal club that you can go along to. This will help you get an idea of what kind of research appraisal is useful in your area.

A lot of this chapter sounds incredibly complicated, and it is. Many students and midwives cover the basics and play to their strengths, whatever those happen to be. If you're up against it and just need a quick way of understanding what kind of research you're looking at, Trisha Greenhalgh (2019: 47) recommends identifying:

- the specific intervention;
- what it was compared with;
- what outcome was measured.

These should help you identify the type of trial. You could also consider:

- the size of the sample;
- where the participants came from;
- what was the treatment/intervention;
- the duration of the follow-up;
- the completeness of the follow-up;
- any statistical tests used.

You would then have a fair estimation of what was going on (Greenhalgh 2019: 54–9).

How much time to spend on appraisal

Your approach to research appraisal will differ depending on your task. If you are writing a long assignment as part of a research module, and you have lots of time allocated to the project, you might be able to go slowly, remind yourself of the literature around the subject, unpack the results and do a refresher on the statistical tests used. If you're checking a new piece of research between shifts, you might be just looking for the basics like peer review, common-sense issues with the methodology and whether there are any published responses to the study.

If you find yourself writing an assignment on one particular kind of research I'd suggest getting a really specific book on the subject, as there's such a lot to be understood about each method. You can often access e-books remotely through your university library for this. As we discussed in Chapter Two, it's challenging to get lots of thoughts about different pieces of research into one single piece of writing, but it's the compare and contrast stuff that will get you high marks. Sara Wickham suggests making a table that compares different studies, as including this kind of resource in your essay can be a great way to get high marks. See her book *101 Tips for Planning, Writing and Surviving your Dissertation* (Wickham 2015).

Even if you're writing a dissertation or another long and complex piece of academic writing, I'd suggest you don't have to reinvent the wheel. Look at the conclusions of meta-analysis studies and opinions from experts. There are always going to be professionals who have spent their whole careers looking at a topic. While you still need to think it through yourself, getting their opinions can be a great help.

Every so often I see a researcher has written a blog post on a piece of midwifery research. I'll dig out the trial and try to come to some conclusions before reading the expert analysis in the blog. I did this with a recent study on caffeine consumption and the risk of stillbirth (Heazell et al. 2021). I went through it carefully and noted some of my questions. When I read the analysis posted by Sara Wickham and Amy Brown I was pleased that I had roughly 60 per cent of the same concerns as they had (Wickham 2022). That's a good effort for me at this point.

To conclude

Keeping up to date with well-designed research is helpful as it points the way to better care. As you progress through your course your ability in this area will become more sophisticated and your assignments will become more research focused. As you move forward in your career, your research critique skills might mean you're able to write guidelines or make changes to an area of midwifery care which you feel passionate about. And if a woman or birthing person in your care wants to make a choice that lies outside medical or midwifery guidelines, being able to assess the validity of the relevant research may at times be a powerful tool in helping advocate for their wishes.

Remember that like with all skills, first, we imitate, then we innovate. Innovation doesn't tend to be a thing undergraduates do: that's what a Masters or PhD is for. I have a go and expect to get some things wrong but to come to some interesting and useful conclusions along the way.

7 Your First Midwifery Placements

Introduction

In this chapter we'll cover what will be expected of you during your first placements; a very exciting time. We'll start with the standard requirements of most midwifery workplaces, and move on to gaining basic midwifery skills. We'll also consider navigating professional relationships with staff and clients, including how it feels to try out your new skills on real people, and how to offer excellent care, even during difficult situations such as bereavement. Finally, I'll cover things you can do to take care of yourself, working towards keeping your enthusiasm and compassion afloat in an intense environment.

Uniform/work clothes

It's likely that as a student midwife you'll have to follow a uniform policy. Some of these rules come from a solid infection control basis, and some are from the cultural heritage of healthcare (Birmingham City University 2019; Durant 2015). It's likely you will need to wear a standard-issue uniform, tie up your hair so it doesn't reach your collar, be bare below the elbows and wear shoes that are low heel and washable. The bit about the shoes is good advice; it's likely you will get them covered with amniotic fluid, blood or vomit at some point. You will also be asked to take off any jewellery, fake nails/nail polish, fake lashes or heavy make-up.

You can check out the midwifediaries.com article 'Midwife Uniforms: Professional or Opressional' (Durant 2015), and from the title you can figure out my take on things. Having said this, I do wear a uniform and uniform policy is not something I tend to challenge, partly because I think it would be an uphill struggle and partly because I quite like my uniform. I'm also frequently asked about whether midwives can have tattoos; I've never heard of a student being refused a place on a course because of a tattoo, but of course, if you had an offensive one that would be an issue. If you need to challenge anything about your clothes or appearance in practice, the podcast 'In Conversation with Fatimah Mohamied' is a good place to start amassing information, since this is what this midwife needed to do (All4Maternity 2020).

A list of items for placement

It's not necessary to buy much for placement but the following were recommended by students and midwives in the online community I run.

Box 7.1: Student and midwife recommendations on what to buy for placement

1. A fob watch.

2. An A–Z notebook, to write down anything from how to use software, to blood bottle colours, to where things are in the storeroom. These notebooks are useful because you can write under alphabetized headings.

3. A pencil case to keep your ID and name badge, pens, fob watch, etc., in so you don't have to scrabble around in your bag at the beginning of a shift.

4. A small midwifery dictionary or handbook – optional.

5. A stethoscope – also optional. Having your own may be a good idea if you're prone to ear infections (do clean hospital ones before you use them).

Initial placements

I promise that getting good at the basics and having a respectful manner with clients and staff is all that's needed for your first placement to go well. Your practice supervisor will take the lead in most situations, and you'll pick a lot up via osmosis.

Have a look at Table 7.1, in which I've put together some of the skills that you will start to have a go at.

Table 7.1: Skills on placement

Initial skills for new student midwives	Further skills for junior student midwives
Knowing how to pull the emergency buzzer/call for help – even if you don't have to do this on your first placements, it will happen sooner or later and knowing how to summon immediate help is important.	Care during births! Initially, you will need lots of support. Care will include auscultating fetal hearts with a sonicaid and pinard, and facilitating water birth.
Hand washing – do this before and after client contact. We're all pros at this since Covid but perhaps watch a video on handwashing, paying attention to the areas that are commonly missed.	Breastfeeding/chestfeeding support – lactation support is worthy of a whole other degree but knowing the basics is helpful.
Knowing how to start a CTG (cardiotocograph, which we use to monitor fetal heart when continuous monitoring is needed), and knowing when a CTG looks extremely alarming (perhaps look up 'fetal bradycardia' in a CTG guide). Bonus points: knowing that position changes can help a fetal heart recover; usually this means helping a client into the left lateral position. You won't be expected to handle this situation on your own especially when you're new, but having an idea about management will be beneficial.	Being able to talk to clients on the phone, knowing what to ask to be safe, where to document and reporting to a practice supervisor with any concerns.
How to perform urinalysis, and knowing when results would warrant referral and/or the sending off of a sample.	Palpation skills, measuring fundal heights to check fetal growth, and starting to work out fetal position.
Completing and recording basic observations for adults: blood pressure, temperature, pulse, respiration rate, oxygen saturation. Reporting back to registered staff members if they are abnormal.	Knowing how to check a placenta is complete and has three vessels (two arteries and one vein).
Completing and recording basic observations for babies: temperature, heart rate, respiration rate. Reporting back to registered staff members if anything is abnormal.	
Taking manual blood pressures for adults using a stethoscope and sphygmomanometer, and knowing when to do this, for instance, if a client has hypertension.	
Beginning to join in with normal, routine antenatal and postnatal examinations, and questions that are part of them. For instance, if a client is antenatal, we will almost always ask if they feel their baby is moving normally, and that they do not have any pain, vaginal bleeding or other vaginal loss. If they are postnatal, we will almost always ask about how often their baby is feeding, and whether they are having wet and dirty nappies. We will also check babies for jaundice.	

Initial skills for new student midwives	Further skills for junior student midwives
Understanding what midwifery drugs are for and how they're given; knowing where to dispense oral drugs from and how to do this under supervision; perhaps taking part in giving subcutaneous and intramuscular injections (extra points if you can rattle off the 'five rights': the right patient, the right drug, the right dose, the right route, and the right time.) Knowing how to use the phone to bleep members of the multidisciplinary team (many of my practice supervisors had a good laugh at my initial attempts as I got through to the wrong person. These days when joining a new trust it's one of the things I'll insist on staff showing me, and I'll write the process out step by step in my A–Z book).	

Rapid learning

If you're anything like me, just because you've correctly performed a skill a few times doesn't mean you know it for life, and just because you've understood a concept or learned a new word today does not mean you'll have a handle on it for tomorrow. This can be really frustrating, but I do have a few tips on how to learn things more quickly.

Box 7.2: Tips for rapid learning on placement

1. Find an excellent source of clinical information from which to make notes. In the UK this might mean the 'Prompt' obstetric emergencies guide (Winter 2018), or perhaps 'The Motivational Midwife' YouTube channel (Jones 2021).

2. Make your own 'lot to remember cards', using clear plastic holders made for conference IDs, which you can find online. You just have to cut the paper to size. Use these for things you'll need all the time, like phone numbers, how to use software, parameters for normal observations and so on.

3. Use Anki or another electronic flashcard app which you can keep on your phone. Use this for more detailed notes, like facts from guidelines, screening information, what to put on an epidural trolley to set it up for an anaesthetist, etc. This way you'll have an evidence-based method for revising information you learn on placement, which is also keyword searchable.

4. Always think through what your care plan might be, even if you don't feel ready to suggest it out loud. You can also write out clinical scenarios and mark them, or do this as a group exercise with other student midwives.

5. To think through a possible care plan, use the SBAR tool, which is the framework many healthcare professionals use to communicate. This stands for Situation Background Assessment Recommendation.

Further information on midwifery skills

Blood pressure

Do you know what blood pressure actually is? Being able to explain it in case a client asks you is a great idea. To quote the writer Bill Bryson (2019: 115):

> The two phases of a heartbeat are known as the systole (when the heart contracts and pushes blood out into the body) and diastole (when it relaxes and refills). The difference between these two is your blood pressure. The two numbers in a blood pressure reading – let's say 120/80, or "120 over 80" when spoken – simply measure the highest and lowest pressures your blood vessels experience with each heartbeat. The first, higher number is the systolic pressure; the second, the diastolic. The numbers specifically measure how many millimetres of mercury is pushed up a calibrated tube. High and low blood pressure can indicate different medical conditions.

Blood pressure was first measured in millimetres of mercury because doctors needed a substance that was a dense fluid. When you take manual blood pressure, you occlude blood flow through a patient or client's arm using a small rugby ball-shaped pump that inflates a cuff. This tallies with a gauge that measures pressure in millimetres of mercury (mmHg).

You then listen with a stethoscope as you slowly decrease the air in the cuff, noting when blood starts to flow again. This sounds like a knock. This first sound is the systolic blood pressure reading. As you keep listening, the sound will turn into a whooshing sound. Once the whooshing sound stops, this is the diastolic blood pressure reading.

Manual blood pressures tend to be more accurate than the ones taken by machines.

Pinard auscultation

A pinard is a trumpet-shaped stethoscope that you can use to auscultate a fetal heart. Though it's easier to use an electronic sonicaid, especially if you're new to midwifery, pinards offer a skilful way of assessing a fetal heart. A pinard can:

- Help you check the findings of palpation as the most likely spot to hear a baby is through the fetal shoulder, i.e. you have to be more particular about where you put a pinard, as opposed to a sonicaid.
- They are a good tool to have if all the sonicaids are in use.
- They can offer a more reliable estimate of a fetal heart considering they are not prone to doubling the reading or other quirks of electronic auscultation methods.

There are some great tips in a resource called 'Pinard Wisdom', which can be found on Dr Sara Wickham's website (2018).

Placement sign-off books

Placement sign-off books can be difficult to navigate and if you're anything like me it can take several passes before you understand what you're being asked to do. (Please forgive me if you're reading this and you're someone who puts these books together; they must be hard to compile and need frequent additions and amendments as legal and trust guidelines change!)

I like to know the direction I should be going in and so if I were training today I would make a list of my own aims using a project management app. I use Trello, which is free, but I'm sure there is lots of other free software around that is also good. This is not about writing out every proficiency in your own words; some of these skills, such as showing kindness and respect, might not be on your own list because they should be signed off incidentally as you offer compassionate care. Your list should be more about knowing what kind of learning opportunities to look out for in practice. You can see an example at the end of this chapter.

About once a week, scan, photocopy or (my preferred method) photograph and upload your documents into a file so if you get your bag nicked or otherwise lose all of those precious signatures, you have a back-up. I know this is a bit of a drag but I used to do it with the TV on in the background. These days if I'm backing up a document I have a workflow using my webcam to make it really easy. You should also do this with timesheets. If you have an electronic sign-off document, in theory this will save you the backing up job, though you may have to talk practice supervisors through how to submit their feedback.

Practice supervisor relationships

One model of learning that I find helpful to consider is Kurt Lewin's 'change cycle' (David 2013). This is essentially a process of unfreeze > change > refreeze. To learn, you need to thaw out and begin to realize there's something you don't know. The learning comes from the disequilibrium and discomfort of 'change'. After you've changed, you freeze again so you can use your new knowledge from a place of stability. Some of the best practice supervisors I've come across will constantly think about and update their practice, taking prompts from students as cues to 'unfreeze'. But especially if your placement area is incredibly busy and your practice supervisors are having to firefight to provide care, they are, by necessity, in the 'freeze' stage. This might contrast with how you're feeling as everything is new.

This model might help you understand your feelings and how to navigate the practice supervisor/student midwife relationship. Also, you might be interested to know that there is a lack of clear evidence around the best components of a teaching relationship. Some researchers say if a relationship is working then there's no need to unpack it and work out why (Woolnough and Fielden 2017: ch. 7). Others say it would be good to have more information around what works, in order to maintain consistency of the level of teaching on offer. But if you think about it, this is a very complex human relationship, so doing research or being prescriptive about what should happen is pretty hard. The best way of coping with all this might be a policy of not judging either you or your practice supervisor too harshly; you will be trying to build a professional relationship and fulfil your respective roles in fast-moving, high-stakes practice situations.

Peer support

I'm very interested in the way students and midwives are using WhatsApp groups for professional support. Obviously, you have to be careful and maintain client confidentiality, and the other rules set by your university/trust, as with any kind of social media. But I'm convinced there is top-notch support going on via WhatsApp. Peer support might also mean asking your student colleagues for guidance or ideas on placement. See more about this in the next chapter.

While we're talking about social media, this can be a great way to find information and be pointed in the direction of up-and-coming research, reports, conferences and so on. Just don't get overwhelmed, there's a lot out there and it can be a bit of a timesink. I went through a stage of trying to follow everyone, but these days I just follow my interests or use social media search facilities to find what I'm interested in. I try to stay active on a couple of platforms and have benefited from sharing and receiving ideas, and the small group of moderators who help run my Facebook group challenge me and keep me looking at the best available evidence. These kinds of online relationships are invaluable.

Mental well-being

There are a few basics that are a good idea to cover when working as a student midwife. When you're working long hours with a physical component, making sure you are well supported by nutrition can help ringfence your energy. Diet is a very personal thing but many midwives I've talked to have found intuitive eating to be a helpful concept (Reshr and Tribole 2020). While we're on this topic, critically appraising evidence around obesity and diets for both ourselves and clients is a constructive exercise. Dr Sara Wickham's blog is a good place to start learning about this (2022).

Your sleep needs as a student midwife are critically important to honour wherever possible. Shift work is challenging. Have a look at the following ideas from students and midwives on managing your sleep around shifts or on-calls, but bear in mind if your sleep is becoming a perpetual difficulty, seeing a specialist can be helpful (Romiszewski, 2021).

Box 7.3: Sleep tips from midwives and students

1. Put up blackout blinds or you can get really nice silk wraparound masks, and use soft silicone earplugs that mould to the shape of your ear.

2. Use melatonin, a hormone that helps control sleep; see your GP for a prescription.

3. Read a reassuring book before bed; fiction can be great for escapism.

4. Try a hot or cold bath before bed, see what works.

5. Eat a small meal before bed (peanut butter on toast, porridge, something that will digest slowly and keep your blood glucose steady).

6. Eliminate or limit caffeine at least six hours before bed.

There are also certain evidence-based activities that will help you look after your mental health. There are breathing exercises which can be good for reducing anxiety, or if you can't find anything that feels right, singing under your breath can have a similar effect. Meditation can help with controlling stress and there is evidence to suggest regular guided sessions can prevent occupational burnout, even for healthcare professionals (Kunzler et al. 2020; Van der Reit et al. 2015).

Beyond this, there are so many midwives, including myself, who've needed a stretch of psychotherapy, and many trusts have a free counselling helpline. There are also various professionals in the birth world who provide paid-for coaching, which can be very helpful (Woolnough and Fielden 2017). Whether you do it with help, or on your own, it's worth identifying what your boundaries are and how to uphold them, as it's so easy to slip into the 'culture of coping' (Kirkham 2007).

Creativity is also an evidence-based way of caring for yourself, as making things can keep you afloat (Brown 2010). Writing has a particularly strong evidence base behind it (Pennebaker 1997). There's a good talk you can find on YouTube called 'Burnout' which has a reference to 'taking anger and knitting it into adorable slippers made of rage' (Nagoski and Nagoski 2019), which I'm sure lots of midwives can relate to! The same researcher who gave the talk has published a book also called *Burnout* which you may want to read (Nagoski and Nagoksi, 2019a).

What it feels like to learn on real people

Have a look at this quote from a student midwife talking about taking blood for the first time (venepuncture):

> I was terrified to start off with as I hate needing to have blood taken and it makes me feel sick! I was shaking loads and so glad I only needed one bottle. I had to sit and calm myself after doing it. Now, coming towards the end of the first year, I am much more confident and no longer shake or feel sick when I have to do it! I don't even mind hidden veins too much.
>
> **Tikki Hills**

This sounds about right. Trying something on a client or patient for the first time can feel very intimidating. It will get easier with time and exposure, I've never come across a student who continued to hate venepuncture or any other skills they have practised. It can feel awkward to be taught in front of and practice on real midwifery clients but the vast majority of people we look after are lovely human beings who have also been in the position of being students at one time or another. I try to accept clients' assistance without too much fuss, but instead, thanks and grace.

Clients who are labouring

Learning how to work around contractions is important; you need to let people get into any position they want and have the headspace that they need. Blood pressures and other observations should be done in between contractions, as otherwise you'll get a reading affected by the intensity. In most situations, you should also aim to keep any questions for the time between contractions. Sometimes you'll need to read the room and work out whether the person having the baby needs quiet. This might be the case if they're hypnobirthing (in which case, you may need to use terms like 'surge' instead of contraction, see the birth plan or ask their birth partner), but sometimes they will be just 'going with the flow' and coping fine but will not have any spare attention. Knowing how to be quiet and chill is otherwise known as 'holding space'.

Remember whoever you're looking after has a culture and life of their own that might be very different to yours, and perhaps different from how it appears. If it seems right to talk, ask open-ended questions and listen carefully to the answers. You can do an amazing job of this, especially as a new student who might have more time to spend with clients (you can see why many midwives love having students).

Don't forget birthing partners. This will be one of their biggest life experiences and they may also be transitioning to being a parent. Just listening to them and checking in can make a big impact.

Even at this stage in your training, you will be coming across ethical and practical controversies. For example, there are studies that show body odour can provide a source of bonding between mother/birthing person and the baby and perhaps putting a hat on the baby just after birth will interfere with this natural process. But on the other hand, we know that babies are born small and wet and are at risk of hypothermia, which makes them less likely to breastfeed and prone to respiratory and other problems (Lundström et al. 2013). Most NHS trusts I've heard of advise a hat after birth and warm dry towels. What's your point of view? It might not be possible at this stage of your career to change a policy of this nature, and you might not have enough information to decide on your take either way, but it's good to be aware of quite how complex and nuanced every midwifery intervention – even putting a hat on a baby – can be. In university, you might well be encouraged to challenge practice as soon as you can, but to begin with, you might find coming to a solid opinion really difficult. I know I did.

I was reminded of another important part of labour care when I watched a TED talk titled 'A Doctor's Touch' (Verghese 2011); essentially, often the skills we complete for clients are about far more than clinical necessity, and how you carry things out using empathetic contact is a vital aspect of midwifery.

Bereavement

It is essential that you know a little about bereavement care. To offer some important context, 4,533 babies were stillborn or died soon after birth in the UK in 2020, which works out as thirteen families who went through this every day (Stillbirth and Neonatal Death Charity (SANDS) 2021).

The following is based on a midwifediaries.com blog post:

> Back when I was a student, these were the questions I had around bereavement care:
>
> > What if I can't find the right thing to say?
> >
> > What if I somehow make it even worse for them?
> >
> > I'm not religious, what if a family is and I fail them in their needs?

I bet you've spotted the problem already; look at all the 'I' statements! I was making bereavement care all about me. One thing I needed to start doing was sending my attention outwards to the parents and family going through the experience, like shining a torch out instead of in. There was plenty I could have been doing to make the experience even a tiny bit better as like most student midwives; I had empathy and compassion in spades.

Start by actively listening. Active listening isn't just about understanding the meaning, it's about hearing the choice of words, taking in body language, maintaining supportive eye contact if appropriate and trying to work out what's there but is not being said. Midwives should do this in every type of care but if a baby has died it's even more important. If you actively listen you'll be able to match your language choice to the family's and pick up on any specific needs, like cultural traditions, or whether they just want a safe haven to make memories with their baby.

Active verbalizing can be helpful too. This is about validating thoughts and experiences, so if they say 'I feel like this is all my fault' instead of saying 'it's not' straight off, you can echo 'ok, you feel like this is all your fault ...' to show them they're being listened to and this isn't a silly thing to be feeling. Then you can go on to say 'but what's happened to your baby is tragic and is absolutely not your fault'.

However, stay away from 'at least' statements. Even the most experienced of staff can sometimes slip into saying 'at least you got to meet them', 'at least you can get pregnant', or most horrific, 'at least you didn't get to know them before you lost them'. Any attempt to frame things more positively is likely to cause more pain.

Remember, however much your practice supervisor prides themselves on being 'tough' the death of a baby is always a tragedy, so ask them if they're ok. There's plenty you can do in terms of basics, like making sure linen is clean, there are enough pads, drinks and snacks are kept topped up and buzzers are answered promptly. Volunteer to get your practice supervisor a drink or do the clearing up so they can have a few minutes. They might laugh as you're less experienced but caring for all members of your team is always the right thing to do.

Remember the partner. This is so important, whatever their gender. I've heard partners call the death of their baby 'hell on earth'. As a student, you'll often have a bit more time and may be able to make all the difference for them. While care must always have the client at the centre, caring for partners is a huge part of holistic midwifery. Listen to what they have to say. Get them involved in the care of the baby if they want to be, things like dressing them, changing their nappy, taking photos or taking a lock of hair. Treat them as all important, because they are. Talks and other online resources to help you understand further are available from David Monteith, whose daughter Grace died before she was born in 2014, and Chris Binnie, whose little boy Henry also died shortly before birth, also in 2014.

Do your own preparation at home. Spend some time on YouTube looking at the many videos on the topic of infant loss. We're in a privileged time; bereaved parents have made us many resources to learn from, for free. It will be especially useful to see what babies look like at different gestations or who are in poor condition. This experience will help you as it's a shock the first time you see a deceased baby, and when you're caring for parents you want your emotional energy to be spent on them rather than your own reaction. Find something beautiful to comment on. I once looked after a woman who had a traumatic and complicated stillbirth and the baby was in poor condition, but he had beautiful eyebrows and eyelashes. She lit up when I commented on this.

Finally, it's ok to cry. You don't have to be a robot. Crying with parents is sometimes the best care you can offer as it validates what they're going through. Of course, you can't make it all about you and parents should never be comforting you. But showing your emotions is part of building that mutual respect that all midwifery care should be based on.

To quote my friend Chantal who runs the The Foundation for Infant Loss: 'I think if you do not care or feel anything at times such as these, then really you're in the wrong profession.'

At the time of writing there is amazing free training available for student midwives via SANDS, and Beyond Bea Charity.

Further placements

As you progress in your training, perhaps around the second or third year of an undergraduate degree course, you might start to practise or master:

- aseptic technique
- catheterization
- handing over clients to a different staff member
- confidence with vaginal examinations
- high-quality record keeping and skills for very complex care, including for clients who are in high-dependency areas
- complex CTG interpretation
- identifying different kinds of perineal tears
- knowing what to check and how often to do observations for a patient in recovery
- setting up for epidurals and monitoring epidural analgesia
- recognizing abnormal blood results
- understanding of care for complex obstetric conditions like placental abnormalities, pre-eclampsia and obstetric cholestasis
- understanding care for complex medical conditions like diabetes, epilepsy or severe asthma
- complex breastfeeding support
- involvement with obstetric emergencies, knowing how to get the relevant equipment, trolley, etc., into the room, participation in emergencies under direct supervision

- there are also lots of specialist midwife roles and other teams you will need to know about and how to refer to – these cover client needs like safeguarding, physiotherapy, fetal medicine and many more depending on your country and area.

This might look like a daunting list right now but if you keep turning up you'll get it and once you're up and running as a qualified midwife it feels really good to be able to do these things for clients. A student placement goals list might look like the following.

Box 7.4: Student placement goal list

Placement proficiencies to complete

Antenatal examinations under supervision (10)

Postnatal examinations under supervision (10)

Guidelines/documents to read

- Nursing and Midwifery Council Code
- Data Protection Guideline for Trust
- NHS Screening Committee Programmes

Verbal skills to demonstrate under supervision

- Take emergency phone call and refer appropriately
- Talk through Down's, Edwards and Patau's syndrome at 12-week appointment
- Add to conversation in parentcraft
- Identify referral that needs to be made to medical team

Skills to demonstrate under supervision

- Abdominal Palpation
- Sonicaid Auscultation
- Pinard Auscultation

Venepuncture (attempts successful)

- Venepuncture
- Venepuncture
- Venepuncture

Meetings with practice supervisor

- Initial
- 3-week review
- Final

Stuff to ask practice supervisor

- Should I buy a pinard or is there one available?
- Where are the screening leaflets?

Study days before practical skills on placement

- Venepuncture

You'll need a bit of experience of placement before making your list and you may also decide this is process is a little over-engineered for you, which is totally fine.

To conclude

It might help to know that we all make mistakes in practice. There is a video and blog post called 'Student Midwife Fails' on midwifediaries.com which you may find funny and helpful (Durant 2014). We have all made more mistakes than we will admit to, and most of our clients are very understanding as they know we are finding our feet!

And just a reminder that the midwives you're working with *often have no idea how skilled they are.* When it's the water you're swimming in, you don't see it anymore. That means you can end up feeling silly when actually, because all this is new to you, you're the bravest person in the room.

8 Developing Your Clinical Skills

Introduction

Taking a lead in care can be scary, and it might be comforting to know that most students feel intimidated when they are learning. In this chapter we'll cover how you develop into a senior student, and how to meet the leap in expectations. We'll cover documentation, clinical skills, written and verbal handover and how to keep organized on shift. This chapter will also cover the one skill I think is underestimated and will make a big difference in your practice: how to anticipate what might happen next. We'll also discuss where to find support for all of this. We'll end with a comprehensive list of things you will be able to do when you're ready to qualify.

Documentation

Basic principles

Good documentation is essential so that other members of staff can pick up a client's care when you've gone home. It also becomes critically important if in the future there are legal proceedings about care. In addition to these reasons, record keeping should be accurate and in line with your communication to clients, as if they request to see their notes, they should recognize what went on.

What you document will differ depending on where you're practising and whether your notes are digital or not. But there are some basic principles that should help you learn to document well.

1. You should always include the date, time, your name and your role.

2. If you're using a computer, what usually happens is your identity is filled in automatically as part of each entry. If you're working on your practice supervisor's login, you will need to write in who you are at the end of each entry and for best practice, you should use your own logins and get everything countersigned.

3. If you are using digital notes, attend some training on the software package the trust uses, or if this is not available, look out for workflows to fill in or other prompts which can remind you of important tasks.

4. As a student, I used to look at the way practice supervisors wrote particular findings, and make a proforma for my A–Z book which I could then refer back to. With common and important elements of midwifery documentation, I used to put my proforma examples on revision cards so I could memorize them. Have a look at the guidelines for your trust or practice. Or if you're training within an independent group practice, you might find they have some guidance based on the insurance cover or legal support they have.

5. If you want examples, Sara Stewart is an Australian midwife with a blog that features documentation of several key skills, like the findings of abdominal palpation and vaginal examinations (Stewart 2020). Also, make use of social media groups you're part of and ask for advice, though be careful about not sharing confidential or workplace information.

Gaining clinical skills

Just like with previous placements, you might want to go through your placement books so you can prioritize the skills that look the most difficult. I would also give your practice supervisor a heads up about the proficiencies you think are going to be hardest to get signed off.

For example, one proficiency might be something like 'complete and interpret relevant clinical tests when caring for a woman or pregnant person with a complex medical condition'. You might be concerned about getting this signed off because caring for such patients can involve intricate charts, observations and blood results. If you're aware of the challenge, you can then tell your practice supervisor that you find complex care, for say pre-eclampsia (PET), daunting and they can be on the lookout for a patient who has this and is happy to be looked after by a student. You can then gain more experience and see where your weaknesses lie. In my experience, if you have a solid plan to gain experience in a particular area, perhaps even written down, practice supervisors appreciate this and find it easier to support you.

There is also evidence that simulated learning for midwifery is effective (Cooper et al. 2012). You'll have skills lab sessions where you can practise things like palpation, venepuncture and cannulation. Booking a skills lab with a small group of students for some low-stakes practice can help you master manoeuvres for shoulder dystocia or breech birth, along with many other skills.

If you're struggling with a difficult practical skill, for example suturing, one of the most accessible ways to learn is to find a textbook or guideline that is particularly good at explaining it, along with a practical video of a professional undertaking or simulating the task. Break the skills down using the 80/20 rule (what are the top 20 per cent of things you need to remember?) and revise the practical steps. I once practised my suturing skills at home just using a pair of tweezers, a sponge and a needle and thread (though the suturing sets do make things easier, ask your practice development team if they have anything spare you can take home). You could buy an inexpensive mini pelvis and doll to help with birth manoeuvres and you could also make some revision cards or otherwise learn the theory by using active recall methods. See Chapter Three for more on this.

But most skills you learn will be via a practice supervisor, as there are too many to learn at home. Most of us learn by copying an experienced demonstrator and receiving their feedback. The trick is to remain receptive to information, even when it's challenging and you're not getting it right. Failed attempts still very much count towards your learning. Though it's always important to ask and offer true informed choice, midwifery clients do tend to be very patient with learners in my experience.

Your handover sheet

Using your handover sheet to write down information is crucial, especially if you're on a ward where midwifery means supporting women and pregnant people with complex medical needs. I once had a midwife tell me she'd read a study where nurses and midwives on shift were found to gain a new piece of information every two minutes. I've never found the reference, but it feels true to me. I write down everything, make tick lists and check my list against my fob watch many times per shift to make sure I'm not forgetting anything.

Handovers can be set up in different ways but, usually, at the beginning of each shift there will be a group handover where a coordinator tells you about each patient/client in brief. Then you'll go and find the midwife currently caring for the patients/clients you've been allocated to get more information. You might want to use the 'SBAR' tool to organize your handover sheet, by writing 'Situation Background Assessment Recommendation' at the top. Coming back to this basic tool should help you remember things. I write out a proforma summary for each client (I got this from an obstetric textbook years ago, but you may well find something like this set out on printed handover sheets as well).

Box 8.1: Proforma summary for midwifery clients

G

P

Gest

Hb (Iron count)

Blood type

Allergies

Medical history

Obstetric history

Current*:

(* In 'current' I'll note medications given, and I'll start to make a tick list of times of medications and observations, scans and anything else due that shift.)

Let's have a look at how to use this in practice.

I've filled this out pretending I'm a student somewhere in my second year. If some of the medical terms are confusing, use Google or a midwifery handbook. At this point in your training you'd use acronyms and other short ways of writing things but to avoid confusion I've used the whole terms here. Also, it's very likely you would be looking after several clients as opposed to just Zetty, as this is the kind of patient who would be admitted to the antenatal ward instead of being one on one on labour ward. Basically, this is just an example so we can think about how you would take handover and plan care.

Box 8.2: Handover sheet for 1:1 care of patient Zetty Eizak, handover at bedside, on labour ward

Name: Zetty Eizak

G1

P0

Gest: 36+2/40

HB: 109

Blood type: A positive

Allergies: No known allergies

Medical history: nil of note

Obstetric history: scans: no abnormalities detected. Placenta anterior and clear of os. Spontaneous rupture of members 11am clear liquor 19/8/21, contractions 'occasional'. Will be 24 hours post rupture of membranes at 1100

Gestational Diabetes, diet controlled

When we go to see Zetty, we greet her and her partner. As our practice supervisor receives a more detailed handover from Zetty's current midwife, we realize the CTG (Cardiotocograph, which looks at fetal heart rate in reference to contractions) is not currently meeting the hospital criteria of normality. This is a good time to use the SBAR tool ...

Luckily, after 10 minutes the CTG does meet the criteria, there are some good accelerations and all looks well. Phew. So with the help of

Box 8.3: Example of scenario and use of SBAR tool used to think through or write down important information and care plan for patient Zetty Eizak

SBAR tool for Zetty Eizak (Situation, Background, Assessment, Recommendation)

S: Threatened Preterm Labour, no contractions on the CTG currently, describes 'occasional' tightenings for a few seconds every 10 minutes or so

B: Spontaneous Rupture of Membranes 20/8/21 1100

A: Fetal heart recorded on a CTG ongoing from 0630, has not met reassuring criteria as lack of accelerations, reduced variability for 30 minutes. Liquor remains clear.

R: For position change to left lateral and encourage to drink fluids. If CTG does not meet criteria by 50 minutes, for obstetric review and to consider conservative methods, is already cannulated so to start IV fluids. Have let shift leader know.

our practice supervisor, we decide to write out a tick list of tasks we will need to do for Zetty on this twelve-hour shift. In my trust, we use plain paper to write out tasks.

Box 8.4: Task sheet for shift while caring for patient Zetty Eizak

Current:

4 hrly observations:

- 0900
- 1300
- 1700

Medication:

- Oral antibiotics due 0900
- Ask if needs pain relief, tell to buzz if pain gets worse/changes

Blood sugar pre and postprandial:

- Now, then offer breakfast*
- Before lunch
- After lunch
- Before dinner
- After dinner

CTG twice daily, depending on contractions and obstetric care plan:

- AM
- PM

Blood tests:

- Full Blood Count
- Group and Save
- C-reactive protein
- Chase results

---

*If your client has any extra medical needs, or if the CTG is abnormal in any way, it's always worth checking with your practice supervisor before you offer a meal. There might be a reason why the medical team would prefer the client not to eat for now (essentially, if there's any chance the client could end up in theatre, anaesthetists prefer their patients to be fasted). Ultimately, the choice to eat or not is always with the client but offering informed choice usually means being able to tell them what the medical team is thinking too.)

From this you can see the kinds of tasks you might want to keep track of on shift.

Verbal handover

Another skill you will begin to master is verbal handover. This can be daunting, as you may have to give handover to an office full of midwives coming onto the shift, or do it at the patient/client's bedside. When I was learning the art of verbal handover, I can remember saying lots of silly things like describing my patient as '37+7' aka 38 weeks pregnant, or saying 'she is currently going for a bath in the bath'. It's normal, especially if you're new and just coming off a night shift. But usually, best advice is:

- Keep it short and to the point.
- Use the SBAR tool.
- Only mention blood or other results that are abnormal/need chasing for results/require action. If you recite every result it's hard to pick out the important bits.
- Give some indication of what's happening next and a possible care plan.

An underestimated skill: anticipating what could happen next

The one tool that experienced midwives have is the ability to anticipate what might happen next. As a student midwife, trying to predict what might be needed for your client, before it happens, is the one skill I'd say can change your practice immeasurably.

For instance, say you're on a labour ward, and you've been on the night shift. Your client, Tamara, is being induced due to PET. After an Artificial Rupture of Membranes (ARM), Tamara is now in early labour, and has an epidural for pain relief. You have to handover to the day staff because your shift has come to an end.

Box 8.5: Example verbal handover from a student to a midwife on shift change

'This is Tamara. She's having an induction for hypertension and 3+ protein on dipstick picked up by her community midwife five days ago. She has no other pre-eclampsia symptoms apart from oedema in her hands and feet, which is ongoing. She had one normal birth three years ago, after a normal pregnancy. She's now 39+2 with an uneventful pregnancy apart from the pre-eclampsia. When admitted to the antenatal ward she was found to be 3 cm with a favourable cervix, so was ARMd at 1800 yesterday with clear liquor draining and started to contract 2:10 overnight. On 4-hourly observations, her BP ranges from 120/85 to 160/95 and she is taking oral labetalol 200mg BD, which is due at 0900. Her PET bloods have remained deranged but steady since her initial results from day unit five days ago. PCR is slightly elevated. She has a cannula, has started fluids, and an effective epidural was sited at 0600 this morning since her contractions were 3:10 and she was 6 cm. We're also continuously monitoring on the CTG.'

Nice work! Clear, to the point and useful. (But we do use a lot of jargon. I might add 'Tamara, that was in a lot of medical speak, does that sound about right, did you have any questions about what's going on?')

Let's think about another scenario involving Tamara's care. Say you're the one coming onto the shift, you've just taken handover, and you're a final-year student.

Your practice supervisor hasn't met you before and you want to show them the level you're working at, because you're wanting them to sign off some of the harder skills in your placement documents today. You're explaining to your practice supervisor what might happen next. A really impressive piece of communication for a student to have about the plan for looking after Tamara might be the following.

Box 8.6: A more detailed handover from a senior student to a midwife

'We'll need to chase PET blood results this morning and if there are concerns, we'll need a review as the doctors may want to change or add to Tamara's medication and/or, ultimately, expedite birth. Options are to aim for a normal birth with no augmentation, which is what Tamara would prefer according to her birth plan. So for that, we'd hope to be 8 cm or more when we reassess at 10 am. But if contractions remain 3:10, 40 seconds, and labour is not progressing we'll need to let the doctors know who may suggest syntocinon augmentation. A fluid balance chart would be a good idea, and if she can't pass urine on a bedpan we'll need to consider a catheter. We'll also need to keep asking about PET signs and symptoms. We need to do observations at least hourly, and temperature 4 hourly, and block height hourly as well. I noted the last BP was 145/90, so I'd like to recheck that as the first thing we do so we can let the doctors know if it's rising. They may want to give the 9 am labetalol early. If there are concerns about the CTG or anything else we'll also need a review so changes in medication or a decision about expediting birth can be taken. Of course, we need to be talking to Tamara and her partner about all of this, how she's feeling, her gut instinct about this birth and baby, her pain level and anything we can do to promote her privacy and dignity, and her choice. She may want to decline any of this, and at that point we could offer information or refer to the obstetric team, or just document her choices and let the shift leader know, depending on what she wanted and what we felt safe to do within our midwifery role.'

See how in this version the student has a midwifery/obstetric crystal ball and is trying to work out what might happen next and what to do about it? This wouldn't necessarily be the way you would communicate with your practice supervisor; it's a bit much all in one go. It might also be overwhelming for Tamara to hear, it's fairly inaccessible, you would want to make things really understandable for the client. But say you'd popped out of the labour room and your practice supervisor was free for a second outside, or you needed to give a summary to the doctors' ward round, this would be extremely reassuring because you've shown such a high level of understanding of and anticipation for what's happening.

If we're thinking from another point of view, Tamara is now bed-bound because of the epidural (you can get mobile epidurals but they are not common – hopefully they will be one day). The medicalized model of care has taken over, and many midwives and other birth world advocates would say Tarmara's choices are now limited (such situations are well documented and true) (Edwards et al. 2018), but: (a) PET is a medical condition and so asking for obstetric input is what most in the birth world would advise, (b) Tamara may be pleased and reassured that her PET is being managed by the obstetric team and (c) we know that medicalization is a problem so we can keep concentrating on choice and letting Tamara know what the guidelines say, what the evidence says and how other midwifery clients and pregnant people have made choices before. When it comes to fast-paced care in an obstetric unit, my own policy is to do *the very best I can*, while questioning myself, and unless I have cause for concern, assuming the good intent of every member of the multidisciplinary team. (See Chapter Nine for help on what to do if you've witnessed poor practice or something else concerning.)

If you're feeling a little overwhelmed by all this, me too! You can use this chapter to work out what to do next but experience is really the only thing that will help you develop these skills. One study I found on improving performance looked at self-talk and how this can be of benefit for athletes. Water-polo players had greater success with accuracy and distance if they were using motivational self-talk (Hatzigeorgiadis 2004). I'd argue that midwifery is just as demanding as an athletic sport, perhaps more so.

Other important clinical skills

Breastfeeding/chestfeeding

Breastfeeding/chestfeeding support is so important. You may have had some teaching already but the type of support we give in the NHS is limited by the time we have for each woman or postnatal person. I've met lactation consultants with so much knowledge – it's a career in its own right. You might want to try and attend a conference on breastfeeding/chestfeeding, organize one for your university (I know, bit of an ask) or at least have a look at some extra resources. Look at the Unicef Practical Skills Review forms, as well as Amy Brown's *The Positive Breastfeeding Book*. Also the *Pinter and Martin* books by Amy Brown, *Why Breastfeeding Matters* and *Why Tongue-tie Matters* (I found these via interviewing Shannon McGill-Randall, an infant feeding coordinator (2021)).

Understanding practice supervisors

It is important to note the exceptional load on midwifery practice supervisors. As you get further through your placements, you are moving towards qualification, and the task of signing students off to enter the register is a weighty one. I remember first becoming a practice supervisor for senior students and suddenly realizing that being relaxed about a student's practice is a really hard thing. It's a constant debate about how much of the client's care to offer to the student's autonomy and whether that's something that's fair on the client and something I can be legally and professionally accountable for. However, I do think it's easier to be a practice supervisor as opposed to a student. My enjoyment of midwifery definitely increased as I went from senior student, to newly qualified, to band 6. Perks for practice supervisors include seeing how far their student has come and being reminded about some of the foundational challenges of midwifery. And students are so incredibly helpful, they are part of the workforce, as you know. But just to remind you why practice supervisors might act a bit tense sometimes, be patient with us, we're trying too.

Peer support

Many studies have found that peer learning can increase confidence levels. I think it's very normal to worry that your student colleagues appear to be more able than you, but in reality there will probably be little between you. Even if you do have student colleagues who are developing faster than you, use them; student peer support is where a lot of the best learning takes place, so don't be afraid of asking for help (Zwedberg et al. 2021). Vicarious experience from role models who are from a similar background and age, and who have succeeded after difficulties is thought to be best, so if you can find someone like this, watch them to see how they do things. Also, if you are processing a particular event from practice and are ashamed of what happened (this happens to all of us) know that shame can short circuit your ability to problem solve and react (Brown 2010). The feeling will be much easier to deal with if you are able to tell someone what's happening and receive empathy. If this is in the form of peer support make sure you choose the person very wisely; my cohort were brilliant but there were only one or two who were similar enough to me to understand the panicked overthinking inner world that I was dealing with. Every time someone confides in me and asks for support I find it a privilege and there are many students and midwives who are eager to help in this way.

The skills you should have by the end of your training

These skills will differ depending on where you are in the world and what kind of resources you have. But to give you an idea of the level you're aiming for, when you qualify you should be able to do the following:

- Support informed consent, and advocate for a client's wishes using evidence-based information.
- Run antenatal and postnatal clinics.

- Have pharmacology knowledge and experience in safely administering drugs, and an understanding of the legal framework for administration and supply of medications.
- Take the lead in caring for a client during a home birth.
- Undertake vaginal examinations, and be confident about your findings.
- Have comprehensive discussions with the coordinator in charge of the shift and with the medical team.
- Have excellent CTG interpretation skills and know how and when to refer.
- Take the lead in caring for a client during induction of labour including oxytocin augmentation.
- Take the lead in caring for a client who has a complex condition like diabetes, pre-eclampsia or other high-dependency needs.
- Take the lead during births of all kinds, including working with the multidisciplinary team during instrumental, caesarean and multiple births.
- Be involved in bereavement care showing expertise and sensitivity.

As you progress through your training, and upon qualification, you will be expected to summon help, initiate emergency care and function as a member of the team during:

- adult resuscitation, with obstetric focus
- bradycardia
- severe pre-eclampsia, eclampsia, eclamptic seizure
- postpartum haemorrhage
- shoulder dystocia
- cord prolapse
- breech birth
- uterine inversion
- newborn resuscitation.

I hope some of these will never happen to you; for instance, adult resuscitation is something I've only been involved with once (and it was not the client, it was her grandparent). But knowing how you'll deal with these should they occur is important. You will likely participate in skills drills as part of your practice when you're qualified. I'm not sure many midwives are really that comfortable with an eclamptic seizure since it comes up so infrequently. Hence the skills drills.

If you're just beginning to take a lead role, say about halfway through your final year, it would make sense to use the 80/20 rule here. Ask yourself, which are the emergencies you see most frequently, and what would it take for you to be able to be lead midwife throughout?

There are nine emergencies listed, so if we take 80/20 to be true, that's, um, 1.8 emergencies we'll need to be good at. So rounding up to two, you're probably looking at postpartum haemorrhage and bradycardia as the emergencies that happen most frequently. If you know how to be part of the team in these emergencies you're doing well and will be gaining skills and experiences which will transfer to other emergencies. Probably newborn resuscitation and shoulder dystocia would be next on my list. Having a strategy will make it much less overwhelming, as you can't learn everything at once.

Final thoughts

Never forget the client at the centre of your care. I think it's brilliant that we have midwives who can offer sensitive, respectful, informed-choice driven care and high-level medical skills at the same time (though I do think we should be paid a lot more). You may find that you want to specialize in physiological midwifery, where things are more about uncomplex care, and once you qualify, you can pursue a role with a home birth team or a birth centre or transition to working as an independent midwife. But most midwifery jobs will require you to have a certain level of obstetric skill, and you will have to prove yourself proficient in these areas to move on.

It's also worth noting that we all make mistakes and I frequently thought I wouldn't make it through my training. But I wish I'd been less prone to stress and burnout. In many ways, I'm probably the wrong person to talk to about success. I want you to be well and whole, whether that comes with an exceptional performance or not is a different question. But for what it's worth, I believe if you hold your placements lightly you'll be more able to work out what kind of midwifery you want to practice. Remember the attrition rate for student midwives in the UK is at least 30 per cent (Astrup 2018), so think about the long game and look after yourself out there.

From Cardiff University's *Preparation for Practice Placement Handbook* (2017) your checklist for being an exceptional student midwife involves being:

- enthusiastic and committed
- proactive
- willing to learn
- open to constructive feedback.

And if you can achieve those all or most of the time, you have my deep respect!

9

Advocacy, Activism and other Workplace Challenges

Introduction

In this chapter we'll think about some of the challenges in midwifery and where they came from. We'll then cover some strategies to help you advocate for your clients and think about two areas of activism and how you can contribute. This chapter goes on to over bullying, whistle-blowing, grief and mental well-being. These topics are heavy but midwifery is one of the most intense professions I've come across and I know when I was training I would have appreciated transparency. I hope these resources will help you if you've hit a rough patch and will remind you that you're not alone. These issues are mostly from a UK perspective; there will be other factors to take into account in different parts of the world.

Our history and where our challenges come from

There's a brilliant book called *Supervision of Midwives* (Kirkham 1996) which features a discussion of UK lay midwives working around the time of the 1902 Midwives Act. These midwives had no formalized training route and instead learnt from each other and their clients. They were often regulated by the church. When inspecting lay midwives, Medical Officers from the newly formed Midwives Board reported being 'astonished' by lay midwives' 'practical knowledge' and 'self-reliance' and at least one study of the time found that care provided by these working-class, experienced midwives was safer than that of physicians (Heagerty 1996: 17). Unfortunately, many lay midwives were struck off for dubious reasons, like being spotted out drinking (I would have been struck off), having an untidy house (struck off for sure) and in one case, a midwife was recorded as attracting disapproval as she was 'found to be engaged in killing a pig' (Heagerty 1996: 17). Most of these midwives were from financially poor backgrounds and possibly kept animals for meat as part of smallholdings. I doubt very much that the Midwifery Inspector in attendance did not eat sausages. It was more that what these midwives got up to offended middle-class sensibilities, which was an issue as midwifery became governed by middle- to upper-class nurses who were deferential to an increasingly powerful medical profession (Heagerty 1996: 16).

The Midwives Act was put in place in part to provide 'respectable employment for middle class women' and to make sure working-class midwives and clients 'conform[ed] to the values and behaviours considered appropriate for them by their social betters' (Heagerty 1996: 13). Although the original plan was for every midwife in the UK to complete training in order to be licensed, when it came to it, lay midwives had to be invited onto the register too or there wouldn't have been anywhere near enough cover for births. 'Trained' midwives were growing in number, and generally saw the presence of lay midwives on the register to be an 'insult' (Heagerty 1996: 15), but lay midwives still attended the bulk of cases and held most of the midwifery experience.

There's a lot to think about when studying the period around the Midwives Act and our early professionalization. For example, some dismissals were justified, and many trained midwives were struck off too. Check out the *Supervisors of Midwives* book for more. But the point I want to make is that even from the beginning, we were a group of professionals working on the back of a staffing crisis.

Midwifery changed again when royal obstetrician John Peel wrote a report on maternity care in 1970. This suggested there should be provision for all births to take place in hospital (Drife 2016). Almost overnight the suggestion was enacted, birth was taken out of the home, and domiciliary midwifery services suffered (Drife 2016). Cut to midwifery in the modern day, and we are two thousand midwives short (Royal College of Midwives (RCM) 2022a), 96 per cent of midwives have concerns about safe staffing (RCM 2022b), midwifery supervision has been taken out of statute and resources are decided upon by a mainly male-led government (Watson et al. 2022). It may be helpful to think about whether our origins have led to this ongoing state of affairs.

It is also important to identify which voices which have gone unrecorded. I assume that our historical workforce included midwives who were Black and brown since I know that Jamaican nurse Mary Seacole set up a hospital during the Crimean War, and expert Black nurse Annie Brewster managed wards in London in the late 1800s (Queen Mary University of London 2021). However, I can't find any records of Black or brown midwives working in the UK around the time of the Midwives Act. I also couldn't find any records of LGBTQIA+ midwives but given the legal history of this group of people, this is not surprising. It may be helpful to think about how all of the above has led to NHS midwifery care being designed for white, cis-gender, heterosexual women, and the implications of that for clients who do not fit into this category. I have found it necessary to pursue education in order to increase my ability to provide equality of care.

In terms of understanding other power structures which have created challenges for midwives, I have learnt a lot from reading Professor Jo Murphy-Lawless, a sociologist working at the School of Nursing and Midwifery, Trinity College, Dublin. One aspect of Murphy-Lawless' career has been starting the project The Elephant Collective, to remember maternal lives lost unnecessarily, including Bimbo Onanuga and others. Her investigations had a key role to play in securing Ireland's full involvement in the Confidential Enquiry process which investigates maternal/perinatal death in the UK. I have questions about why maternal/perinatal mortality in Ireland was not being satisfactorily investigated for so many years when the UK system was the gold standard globally, and so close geographically (Murphy-Lawless 2019: 133–41). This, combined with the scant options for home or midwife-led unit birth, and the only recently resolved lack of access to termination of pregnancy services, forms a pattern that 'the lives of these [Irish] women simply don't matter very much' (Ingle and Murphy-Lawless 2019). The impact of colonialism is also something I needed to know about while working as a midwife in New Zealand, especially when working with Maori clients. You can't serve midwifery well if you don't understand the history of the area you're living in, how 'power makes itself felt' and how different parties might feel about that (Ingle and Murphy-Lawless 2019).

Modern midwifery and why it's hard to make headway

Mavis Kirkham's seminal 1999 'Culture in Midwifery' paper presents the concept that midwives take on as much as humanly possible, and do so quietly. This might sound like a good thing but it's how oppressed groups of people behave and it's not sustainable. Most midwives believe that we could make some changes by increasing our participation in politics, taking industrial action or simply by putting in more incident reports, but these actions often go against what mid-wives are taught to do, which is to just to keep going without making a fuss (Kirkham 2007). Activism can be exhausting and midwives need to conserve energy to continue to practise. This means midwives may simultaneously feel guilty for not doing enough organized leadership and/or protest, and also overwhelmed by the demands of giving care. The key question is how we put boundaries around well-being while furthering midwifery as a force that can change the world.

Advocacy

A midwife's role includes advocating for the wishes of women and birthing people even when these fall outside medical guidance, and this is a legal requirement which comes from the Human Rights Act (Birthrights 2019). Moreover, the 2015 landmark *Montgomery vs Lanarkshire Health Board* case prompted the following to be added to the law on consent: 'An adult person of sound mind is entitled to decide which, if any, of the available forms of treatment to undergo, and her consent must be obtained before treatment interfering with her bodily integrity is undertaken.'

However, advocacy is not a straightforward process and control and decision making during childbearing are often still in the hands of professionals, as a lot of research tells us (Edwards et al. 2018). Historically, midwifery has struggled to gain the power needed to uphold rights. Learning how to advocate in such circumstances is difficult. Although there will be times you make an enormous difference to the experiences of women and birthing people, it may be best to approach advocacy with your eyes open, knowing that this is a complex and demanding part of midwifery care.

Exploring ways to advocate for midwifery clients

Connecting with advocacy experts

To see how advocacy works, try to work with a midwife who has a reputation for excellence in this area. For instance, in my trust, this would be the manager of the birth centre, amongst others. There may be a formalized process you can get involved in, for instance, a clinic for clients wanting to make decisions outside the guidelines. You may also be able to organize a shift with experienced midwives who have trained as Professional Midwifery Advocates (PMAs). PMAs advocate for women and birthing people, either directly or by supporting less-experienced midwives in an advocacy role (NHS England 2017). You may also be able to shadow an independent midwife in your area. Independent midwives are often booked by clients to help them gain better support for birthing outside guidelines (Birthrights 2017). If you find it difficult to organize this shadowing, you may want to follow a few relevant professionals or organizations online:

- Deborah Neiger is an independent midwife who publishes reflections on Facebook and other channels (2022).
- Mars Lord is a doula and activist particularly addressing racism, and she posts on Instagram and elsewhere (2022).

- Mary Cronk (MBE) was a very experienced midwife who has been interviewed about advocacy. You can find videos of these interviews on YouTube (Cronk 2012; Cronk and Graves 2019).

- It may be worth researching the careers of midwives who have made significant contributions; for instance, Dr Shawn Walker at Kings College London has developed the role of Breech Specialist Midwife (Breech Birth Network 2016); Becky Reed championed one of the first midwifery continuity of carer models available in the modern NHS (Association of Radical Midwives (ARM) 2017).

- Birthrights is a charity which offers legal advice to help champion evidence-based care, via their website.

Another good way to find professionals doing this work is to join a local organization committed to supporting the rights of clients. In the UK this might mean the Association of Radical Midwives (ARM) or the Association of Improvements of Maternity (AIMS).

The BRAIN acronym

In time-pressured and fast-moving care situations, it can be difficult to talk about options in a comprehensive way. The 'BRAIN' acronym is a way to structure your ideas and help clients with decision making. I first saw this on Dr Sara Wickham's blog (2017).

> What are the Benefits (of this course of action)?
> What are the Risks?
> What are the Alternatives?
> What does my Intuition say?
> What if we did Nothing?

For instance, say a client is wondering whether to take some paracetamol for pain relief in labour. We could help them think through their choices. Using BRAIN to prompt us, our conversation might look something like:

What are the benefits? Hopefully, some pain relief to get to a later stage of labour without having a bigger intervention like an epidural.

What are the risks? Probably low, but actually, paracetamol is a prostaglandin inhibitor, so we perhaps don't have enough evidence to say it isn't going to interfere with labour (The Undercover Midwife 2015).

What are the alternatives? Things like massage, a TENS machine or using water in the form of a pool, bath or shower. There may also be some kind of oral opiate pain relief that your trust may offer, which will usually come with side effects like sleepiness, nausea and vomiting (an anti-sickness drug or 'antiemetic' can help). Although the side effects of oral pain relief tend to be mild, paracetamol might be a better option than an opiate medication as it doesn't cause sleepiness in newborn babies, which can prompt difficulties in them establishing breathing and/or breastfeeding.

What does your intuition say? If the client has mixed feelings about taking oral pain relief at this point, perhaps that's an indication they need more information or it's not the right decision – help them think this through.

What if we did nothing? This would be a safe decision to put off, perhaps a natural decision-making point will appear and feel best for the client.

As you progress in your training, you may be able to use the acronym to help clients make decisions about complicated situations such as choosing between a home or hospital birth.

Suggestions from AIMS

Advocacy can feel like a lonely task; to quote my friend and mentor Joy Horner, 'it is such a difficult job for those who care'.

I recently I attended a workshop on informed choice run by AIMS. Connecting with other birth workers was welcome support. I learnt the following, which may be helpful in supporting a client's informed choices.

- If you have a client who has made a particular decision and based on your relationship with them you know they may be experiencing unwanted pressure about this, it can be as simple as reminding them they are their own person and the choice is up to them.

- If you feel your client is unclear on options, you may want to prompt them to ask 'are there any alternatives recommendations?'

- If you feel what you are saying in front of other professionals could be misconstrued as persuading the client one way or the other, you could remind your client of their choices when others have left the room, or if you're a student taking someone to the bathroom, this can be a good moment to remind them that you are their sounding board, and the choices remain with them.

- If your client doesn't understand, offering a quiet, detailed idea of what is happening can help them feel supported.

- Ultimately, your client is an adult who is responsible for their own decisions, you are there to provide information, support and clinical care.

Some particular thoughts for students:

- We need you to pass the course and sometimes the responsibility will be with the qualified members of staff, or in some cases, the doctor; do your best and make sure you qualify because we need you. These situations sometimes come with very hard judgement calls about what you can achieve as a student.

- The workshop ended on a key idea which was: 'There is no need to argue, we all want the same thing which is for choices to be upheld and clients, babies and their families to be happy and healthy.' Working as part of a multidisciplinary team under pressure can be fraught at times, but I think this is a healthy point of view to return to.

(Ashworth et al. 2021)

Activism

Two big areas of activism noted in midwifery over the last few years are around Black and brown midwifery clients, and LGBTQIA+ (particularly trans and non-binary) clients. I'm no expert, but I'll share what I have learnt and signpost to further resources.

Anti-racism

There are so many brilliant resources to help you learn and think about anti-racism. Reni Eddo-Lodge, Christine Ekechi, Nova Reid and Mars Lord, as well as the team from the Association of South Asian Midwives, are my go-to activists in the UK at the moment but there are plenty of fantastic people doing this work globally. I'd suggest looking to history to work out why Black and brown people are suffering far higher rates of mortality and morbidity than their white counterparts. Essentially, the Atlantic slave trade went on for four hundred years and involved more than 12 million enslaved people (Owens and Fett 2019; Ryrie 2015). To think that this has left no mark on our society is a dangerous position for healthcare professionals to take. I'm really interested in the studies that suggest that having Black doctors makes for much safer care for Black clients (Greenwood et al. 2020). This result indicates there are solutions to the problem.

In countries like the UK and USA where detailed data about health and race/ethnicity are collected, it is easy to see the disparity in outcomes between white people and other ethnicities. The MBRRACE report from 2020 found that Black women are five times more likely to die during childbirth, and Asian women are twice as likely to die during childbirth compared with white women (Knight et al. 2020). More recent MBRRACE figures suggest the risk of mortality for Black clients is now down to four times more likely compared to white clients, but actually, this finding is not statistically significant (Knight et al. 2021). In the USA, non-Hispanic, Black women are more than three times more likely to die during the perinatal period (Centres for Disease Control and Prevention (CDC) 2019).

The following are some examples of racism affecting maternity care:

- Women from ethnic minority backgrounds are offered less pain relief than white women, this is something all students and midwives should know about to be able to compensate (Ekechi 2020). It's useful to be aware of history in this area: Black slave women were experimented on without anaesthetic by early obstetrician James Sims. Around the same time, elite white physicians published their views that Black women had 'near immunity from pain during childbirth', a sinister and convenient belief for society profiting from slave ownership. Our ideas about the way Black people experience pain have heritage from this time (Spettel and White 2011).

- Healthcare professionals lack training around the appearance of Black/brown skin. For instance, this makes it difficult to recognize pathological jaundice in newborns who are Black and brown. See *Mind the Gap* for a handbook to help with this (Mukwende, Tamony and Turner 2020).

- There is a lack of diversity in NHS midwives and doctors (Ali 2021; Pendleton et al. 2022), and a lack of diversity in midwifery leaders, especially at board level where influential decisions can be made (Burney-Nicol 2021).

- Black midwives are more likely to be referred to the Nursing and Midwifery Council than white midwives. They are not, however, any more likely to be removed from the register, suggesting they are referred for relatively minor reasons. Both Black and Asian midwives experience lower progression and pay than white midwives (NMC 2020).

There is much more research into racism being undertaken.

In her undergraduate dissertation, my colleague midwife Claire Coomey (2021) drew attention to the process of cultural safety training being standard for New Zealand healthcare professionals. There was originally some negative feedback about the time the concept took to teach compared to other issues but it is now seen as a positive part of training (Papps and Ramsden, 1996), something I can attest to personally. I'd suggest similar training needs to be implemented everywhere. As Dr Christine Ekechi, who is working with RCOG to address race-related mortality, says, 'racial equity education is ... a core skill central to the delivery of equal, safe, and excellent care' (2020).

Many organizations such as Birthrights are calling for further research. In the meantime, I'm proud to say my alma mater De Montfort University is at the forefront with its anti-racist 'decolonising the curriculum' project (De Montfort University (DMU) 2022). *The Good Ally* by Nova Reid, has direct anti-racism instructions for those working in the maternity and perinatal services, and Reid's thoughts on self-care for activists are second to none (Reid 2021). And the outstanding 'Through the Dark Lens' conference, which gathers experts in this area, is one I hope to return to. A commitment to anti-racism is a key way to keep clients safe. If you are not already skilled in this area, I'd suggest taking a course on anti-racism, and if you can, asking your university or hospital to implement some training. (When white people join in with anti-racism movements, we should apologize for having taken so long to show up, by the way.)

LGBTQIA+ rights

The number of people who identify as LGBTQIA+ is increasing globally and the reasons for this are heartening: freedom is contagious (Doyle 2020: 223). In the UK 49 per cent of 18 to 24 year olds now say they are something other than completely heterosexual (Dahlgreen and Shakespeare 2015). Further relevant details include that in 2012, 1.5 per cent of people identified as lesbian, gay or bisexual, rising to 2.7 per cent in 2019 (Office for National Statistics 2021). It's generally acknowledged there is a lack of good quality data on transgender and non-binary people but current estimates are that 650,000 people in the UK do not identify with the sex they were assigned at birth (Women and Equalities Committee 2015).

The following are examples of the unequal treatment of LGBTQIA+ people in the UK:

- Hospital notes and other official forms don't usually have spaces for same-sex couples to fill in details, they will refer to 'mother' and 'father'.
- Transgender and non-binary people currently have no way of correctly referring to themselves on legal documents about parenthood.

● Transgender men who childbear face challenges around being correctly entered onto computer systems and may have to be classed as female to get the proper care. There are reports that blood tests are rejected as the system gets confused if they are labelled as male. Trans people can get left out of current or future screening programmes because their identity is not trackable by current practice databases.

(Examples drawn from the work of A. J. Silver 2017, 2019; Workshop 2021)

There are far more inequality issues than I've listed here, including LGBTQIA+ people facing greater risks of violent crime (Metcalf and Hudson-Sharp 2016; Office for National Statistics 2017).

Another current issue for this group of clients is the controversy around using inclusive terms, for instance, using 'woman and birthing person' instead of just 'woman' when we're writing guidelines or talking to a group of clients whose identity is unknown. Some feel that this detracts from the one arena that women have always owned. However, this group of people have also always been here, we've just erased them for the official narrative at the moment. Professor Lucy Delap, who teaches gender history at Cambridge University, suggests that feminism should be rooted 'in a concept of embodied, gendered practices and material contexts, replacing divisive talk of gender as performance or bio-genetic.' She goes on to write that 'we are likely to see new histories being written that reveal a deeper history of gender nonconformity' (2021: 340). I understand this to mean that we should look at what women are experiencing, rather than what defines a woman and that, also, we all have a lot to learn. I continue to embrace feminism because I think we're all hurt by the patriarchy, but instead of just one 'feminism' I think there are many 'feminisms' and in midwifery, the feminism we're looking for must tackle racism, sexism, classism, ableism, anti-LGBTQIA+ rhetoric and violence, and more.

I have also seen the complaint that transgender and non-binary people are getting a lot of attention and perhaps more common issues like disability, mental illness, birth trauma, etc., are more important to focus on. Firstly, to quote A. J. Silver: 'This isn't trauma top trumps ... inclusion isn't pie, there is always enough to go around if we choose' (2019). Secondly, disabled or mentally ill people also have a gender and sexuality, so they are part of this too. We see identity as rooted in gender and if we're talking about sexuality, to quote researcher Jamie Hale, 'People often assume that just because we're disabled, we don't have any sexuality or any interest in sex whatsoever. It's a form of infantilising us ... there are lots of disabled lesbian, gay, bi and queer [LGBTQIA+] people out there, and we find partners and love the same way everyone else does' (2019). And actually, inclusive language doesn't cost money. In terms of disability, most perinatal services in the UK have a long way to go – think about the wards at your local hospital, are there multiple rooms with ensuite bathrooms that easily accommodate wheelchairs? Probably not. But we should be able to get at least the basics right, including preferred language choices and a good attitude towards clients with additional needs, something which we're not doing so well on at the moment (Birthrights 2019).

The data suggests that midwives will see an increase in the percentage of LGBTQ+ people we look after. Becoming skilled in care for transgender and non-binary people requires far more than getting pronouns and other terms right (though this is a good start).

Take a course run by an LGBTQIA+ activist in the UK. A. J. Silver is my go-to person, and their excellent book 'Supporting Queer Birth' (2022) is now out. Nathan Welch of TransMidwife YouTube fame is also hugely useful. If you can, ask your university or hospital to provide training – asking them is a form of activism.

There are of course many other areas in need of midwifery specialists. These include disabilities and learning difficulties and how to support and normalize birth and parenthood for these groups of people; people suffering from addiction and the stigma and lack of funding; women and birthing people suffering from mental illness; mothers and/or parents who are vulnerable to domestic abuse ... If you have an area you are passionate about and you'd like to think about a leadership position in midwifery, brilliant, you're sorely needed.

It will probably take a while to find how best you can help as an individual. For my part, I know I have written this chapter through my own white, heterosexual, middle-class lens, so feedback is always welcome.

Bullying in midwifery

Though there is no one accepted definition of bullying, the work of midwife Dr Patricia Gillen suggests that core components of bullying are that it is a repeated behaviour, it is difficult to defend against and it has a negative effect on the person being bullied. Quoting from Gillen's work (2009, 2021), 43 per cent of student midwives have witnessed bullying and 30 per cent have experienced it. Other researchers suggest the concept of 'civility' is more helpful than the word 'bullying' in clinical practice, as one person's brusqueness is another's bullying (Turner et al. 2018).

Interviewing a midwife psychotherapist was an insightful exercise for me – have a look at the following.

A midwife psychotherapist's perspective

Box 9.1: Midwife psychotherapist Julia Reissmann on bullying

I wonder whether bullying is passed down. That sort of hierarchy structure where students are at the bottom can be really hard. When I trained as a midwife, I'd had proper jobs, I'd worked in homelessness, and had led training sessions. So I had what I thought to be a lot of valid and relevant experience. But when I started in midwifery, it was wiped clean, you're starting from scratch, and you know nothing, you are at the bottom rung. And all you can do is work your way up the hierarchy. And some people come into midwifery with a real desire to facilitate normal birth, to be an advocate, to give the best care possible and they're quite idealistic. And it's a shock when you get in, you think, 'I didn't know it was going to be like this! What about all the books I've read!'

This is what I experienced. Older midwives almost need you to conform, it's very parental. It relates to the idea of the inner critic. When we're student midwives it's like we're children, and the older midwives are like adults. They have to mould us in the same way as they were moulded because otherwise, students are not going to manage in this midwifery world, which is not perfect.

We all do it as parents to some extent. It's like wanting to crush a free-spirited child who just wants to dance all day. And it's like, 'no, you can't do that, you need to get into school and sit down and not move and do what you're told'. And you become really critical. You criticize because you don't want your child to be criticized by other people. This is exactly what we do with our internal critics, by the way.

And I wonder whether there is some of that which goes on in midwifery, you can't just be free, you have to knuckle down. I think that's what's going on, that's the bigger structure.

Unfortunately, you can't create a culture where women are really treated respectfully unless the midwives are treated with respect by their managers, and so on above them.

Most of us know how hard midwifery is going to be, we come in with our eyes open. But just like being a parent or being in a long-term relationship or writing a book, you can't really understand the challenge until you're in the middle of it. Those midwives who are being critical might not be helping you but they do know how to survive in a very hard profession and sometimes you just have to say, god that must have been hard, and take the good things.

Reissmann (2021)

Julia's point about knowing how difficult it has been for those who have been bullied helps me a lot. Also, boundaries are of paramount importance.

Box 9.2: Further strategies and resources for addressing bullying

- Most experts and organizations suggest documenting what is happening so you have something to draw from should you end up needing to take further action, or you need to provide evidence to a senior member of staff; see The Royal College of Nursing Bullying and Harassment diary, found on their website.

- Aryanne Oade, a chartered psychologist, has published recommended books on workplace bullying (2015, 2017).

- See the 'Stop Bullying in Midwifery' Facebook group.

- The 'Midwives Haven' telephone support can be found on the Association of Radical Midwives website.

- Amanda Burleigh, an award-winning midwife who has identified issues for many years now, and Helen Elliott-Mainwaring (2021), who is completing her PhD on this topic, are two other midwives whose work at conferences or in journals is well worth following.

- I personally needed to work out how my own history was contributing to producing an emotional 'allergic reaction' to certain situations. Support from a psychotherapist has had a strong effect on my ability to practise when complex human factors interfere with care.

Bullying targeted towards those in oppressed groups

In terms of bullying fuelled by racism, it is important, though depressing, to understand that 66 per cent of students impacted by racial bias do not raise the issue with their university (Burnett 2021). Obviously, the best course is to report discrimination but I realize you may not be able to. You could get in touch with your student or midwifery union, or contact a senior midwife who you know is attached to a university committed to anti-racism and decolonizing the curriculum. You may also get good support through an activist group.

Similar strategies may be useful if you are experiencing bullying due to belonging to a group who are discriminated against, for example if you are LGBTQIA+ or disabled. Collaboration between activists advocating for these groups of people exists, and similar skills are needed to address such issues, so it may be worth building your support group and hearing from those in the birth world who have faced issues (Lord and Silver 2021).

Whistle-blowing

Hopefully, if you see poor practice, a 'firm, polite challenge', such as saying 'I'd be happy to help you ring for a senior midwife opinion as I feel that's what's needed', would be enough to address the situation (Care Quality Commission (CQC) 2021). However, as a student or newly qualified midwife who is depending on good feedback, this can be difficult (Gillen 2021). If your 'firm, polite challenge' doesn't work or you're not able to do this, you can consider submitting an incident report. These will be assessed by the relevant senior team and can be very useful especially as you don't have to identify individual members of staff. The feedback from the incident report may be communicated to staff via a group email, or another way of spreading information about an issue that needs to be addressed by everyone.

If I were raising something within my trust that came down to a concern about an individual, I might go to a senior member of staff I trusted and ask what kind of protection I was entitled to as a whistle-blower. But it's important not to ignore these things. In the UK there have been recent devastating failures in perinatal care (Independent Maternity Review 2022). I'm aware that catastrophic working cultures due to staffing or other pressures can be unimaginably difficult to navigate as an experienced member of staff, let alone a student or newly qualified midwife.

If you find yourself in the middle of situations you know are unsafe, you might want to consider talking to your union, a local midwifery organization or looking at your local whistle-blowing policy. In the UK there is also a whistle-blowing NHS helpline, as well as the charity Public Concern at Work. Birthrights charity might also be useful. I'm lucky to have a list of experienced midwives to call on, and if I found myself in this position I would contact them.

If you don't feel your concern is being taken seriously, you might have to make a decision to take it to an official body. In the UK this would mean the Care Quality Commission (CQC). There are guidelines on their website you can follow. You may also take the decision to move away from your trust if you feel it's continually unsafe and no one is listening. This is a rare occurrence but we should all be prepared for this as being a midwife means being responsible for lives, so the best course may be to get out and attract attention from there.

Failure

> When I was in my second year, my mentor went out of the room for pethidine. I was standing chatting to the family about pethidine and I didn't notice the 2-minute bradycardia. My mentor came back in, we pulled the bell and laid the woman on her left and it recovered straight away.
>
> My mentor handled it brilliantly with me. After the shift asked how I felt about it, I burst into tears because I felt so awful, and she said that's great because I know you've learnt from the experience now (this is almost 7 years ago now so I absolutely have!)
>
> **Anonymous**

This is such a good example of a positive learning experience, but we can be in the depths of shame when events like this happen. Failure sucks, but I know you want a brave life, or you wouldn't have chosen midwifery. Bravery does not exist without 'uncertainty, risk, and emotional exposure' Brown 2012: xii), and flat-on-your-face moments are guaranteed. Things get a little easier as you begin to realize that you are capable of getting back up again.

If we're talking about final-year placements which are calling into question your ability to graduate or be on the midwifery register, I'm really sorry this is happening. As you approach qualification, the atmosphere of clinical practice can change. As a more junior student, you may have had to be accommodating about putting client care first, which can mean stepping back and observing. But now the spotlight is on you. There is an element of final placements which can feel like driving test conditions. For me, this point of having to continually explain my practice while still being fairly new was much more of a challenge than being newly qualified. Sometimes it helps to realize that individual practice supervisors need to assess you but they can't have a 360-degree awareness of how your practice is going, they just have to make their minds up based on what they see. If you receive criticism, it may well be okay to reflect on the useful parts of feedback without taking it wholesale. In the Facebook group for student midwives that I run there was a feeling of being much more comfortable and competent when being alone with a client. As soon as a practice supervisor steps away, you end up having some agency over the situation and you realize you can do it.

Melissa Newman, midwife and current doctoral student, advises not to let people stop you and recommends that you 'let success be your noise'. As much as I will always strive for an environment where students do not feel they are stopped by anyone, there might be times when you have to take this position.

The following is a quote from an anonymous student in 2018 talking about failing her final placement, but then finding support and qualifying. This is the kind of mentorship the profession is aiming for:

> I think more effective than resilience is kindness, patience and gentleness. In my worst moments, I had kindness poured over me from hearts steadier than my own. I had ears that heard me and allowed me to speak, and many people who were willing to tread a path with me. This, more than anything, helped me to survive, heal and ultimately thrive. I am stronger, not by my own might, but by the strength of those who held me up when I couldn't do it alone.

Grief

This post was put on social media by independent midwife Deborah Neiger (2022) in the aftermath of a tragedy with one of her clients. I don't think I can sum up grief in midwifery any better.

Box 9.3: Coping with grief in midwifery

Sometimes midwifery will deal your clients and you such a hard blow that it feels like your life is forever changed and you are plunged into a dark place ... please be ready for that. In a profession such as midwifery which requires passion, emotional involvement and dedication for you to be good at it, that very same passion, emotional involvement and dedication can bite you in the butt, hard.

Find your people/allies.

Explain your passion and emotional involvement to those around you so that they can somehow understand when it happens.

Build a support network so you can fall back on people who care about you.

Be aware of what you need in terms of self-care in times of distress.

And be kind to yourself. Always.

Also, vulnerability is not a weak point and does not need to be hidden from view at all times.

Mental well-being

I recommend the XOXO talk 'Burnout' (Nagoski and Nagoksi, 2019b) which discusses stress hormones getting stuck in the body and causing harm. The trick is to take a break from whatever is causing you stress, move through the emotion like it's a tunnel and recover a bit before diving back in. It sounds like common sense but this talk was the first time I've heard it described this way. It's also important to discuss suicide. Though we don't have a specific statistic for midwives, nurses were recently found to have a 23 per cent higher risk of taking their own lives compared to the general population (Hughes 2018). Researcher Carolyn Hastie suggests that a culture of bullying and other work issues can contribute to suicidal thinking and action in midwives (1996).

I commend midwife Amity Reed who has written candidly about her attempt to take her own life (2020). I don't have the evidence for my next point but I think responsibility and pressure combined with a caring nature and a lack of agency to make changes can create perfect conditions for suicidal ideation.

If you are experiencing suicidal thoughts or want to hurt yourself, please don't be alone. In the UK and Ireland, a good place to start would be the Samaritans, who are available through phone calls, emails and text messaging. Even if you know you'd never act on your thoughts, it might be sensible and kind to yourself to see a counsellor. I know a lot of brilliant midwives with depression or anxiety who take medication or have ongoing counselling/psychotherapy. Honouring mental health needs is perfectly compatible with an amazing life.

The other thing to mention is that I've run a midwifery community online for eight years now and I can tell you that many, many excellent students take a break in their studies, and the same goes for midwives who need some time away from their career. Midwifery is intense and your health must come first.

> I had a breakdown halfway through my final year and failed a placement because of it. I'll qualify six months after my classmates. I'm now repeating the placement and I've been given buckets of support by the staff I'm working with. No one has judged me – lots of people have contacted me saying similar things happened to them with failing or taking time out for their mental health at some point during the degree. It's a hard job, a hard course, it's a show of good character that you had the sense to press pause and put yourself first.
>
> **Senior student midwife Laura Henry**

To conclude

I mentioned Nathan Welch above. He's a midwife I've known online for a long time and is also a moderator for the Facebook group I run. He once posted the song 'Be More Kind' by Frank Turner (2018) into our mods group, commenting that it was our song, since our first rule is the adapted quote 'always be kinder than necessary, everyone is fighting a battle you know nothing about' (MacLaren 1984). I thought it was going to be a little corny but listening to it, it has exactly the energy needed. Whether it's towards yourself, staff or clients, the lyric that always comes back to me is 'in a world that has decided that it's going to lose its mind, be more kind, my friends, try to be more kind'.

10 Job Applications and Interviews

Introduction

If there's one thing I want you to take away from this chapter it's the following: as a newly qualified midwife you might have real fears about your first job. This is normal, and it's good to talk about this with someone trustworthy. But even if you're feeling wobbly, your job application and interview should focus on your strengths, not your weaknesses. Also, you might be still training, or coming up to a final stretch of exams, and be on your last energy reserves. But I promise you that writing your application can be a quick and confidence-building activity. This is the time to be an advocate for yourself and show your strengths.

This chapter will help you put together a competitive written application, and to give a strong interview performance. I've included lots of examples and tips from qualified midwives who have been through the process. As you read through this chapter, remember how hard you've worked, and how far you've progressed. Try to take confidence from your ability – why shouldn't your potential employer be delighted to hear from you?

Written application skills

There are different kinds of written applications that prospective workplaces can ask you to complete, including personal statements and CVs. A personal statement is exactly what it sounds like: a long-form piece of writing that's all about you and tells your employer what you have to offer. Sometimes you'll need to fill in an application form which is split into different sections like 'description of duties and responsibilities' or which contain specific questions that you are expected to answer, for example, 'What are your reasons for applying for this position?' This is essentially the same thing as a personal statement, just with some guidance to help you structure.

In general, when you write about a skill you've taken from a job description or specification, you should unpack it a little, offering some evidence of your understanding by clarifying why it's important, rather than just repeating the words and phrases. You may also want to describe some of your practice experiences to help you illustrate what you can offer; it's always more powerful to show rather than tell.

Examples of written applications

Have a look at the examples below. Feel free to skip to the kind that's been requested by your prospective workplace, but I've tried to make each example fun to read and worth your time in terms of learning application technique.

Longer personal statements

First let's look at some examples of personal statements that have a longer word count. You might have an unlimited word count, or close to it at 1,000 words or more. Even if your word count is unlimited, I wouldn't go above 1,000 words as most of the staff reading your application will be very busy.

I often find it easiest to learn from what not to do, so with the below statement I've greatly exaggerated some of the most critical errors that can be made.

Box 10.1: A longer personal statement – poor technique

I am applying for the role of Band 5 newly qualified midwife at Danebury Trust because I will soon be ready for employment. I am excited at the prospect of joining the trust and would bring my strong belief in midwifery as a concept. Your Hospitals are the no.1 for my application considering the labour ward, mixed antenatal and postnatal ward, and neonatal unit. I am looking forward to working in each and every area. I am looking forward to qualification so I can be purely practical rather than being bogged down in theory.

My training so far has equipped me for all manner of midwifery care. I have experience with obstetric emergencies like PPH that sometimes need to be managed by the non-senior team in cases where everyone is busy. I will be an asset to the team as sometimes the coordinator midwives can be very overwhelmed, you have to know how to muddle through on your own. I am also very good at communicating with gestures with our clients who don't speak English, as translation services are expensive.

I can also handle it when practice becomes very busy and we have to prioritize care over little things like documentation. I can take and give tough feedback and believe in being honest so people understand which professional is to blame. I am keen to get students the experience they need and feel we do not make as much use of births as we could, especially as women don't generally notice who is in the room at the pushing stage. I do not enjoy postnatal care but really hope I could just work on labour ward.

I found my university lacking in many ways but feel practical midwifery is not about book learning so this will not be a problem. To explain my needs, I have not had many opportunities to practice harder skills like being in theatre, and based on feedback from practice supervisors, my CTG interpretation skills sometimes trip me up. However I know with a preceptorship package, it would be fine.

I have witnessed some poor discussions of care with women that left them feeling belittled, something I would want to challenge as I become more senior. I would be excited to start my career off at your trust, which is where my preference would lie for my first role, given it is within driving distance of my home. As long as my car doesn't break I'd aim to be on time for shifts (though am experienced at working out what's happened if I've missed handover).

I'm being facetious; I don't believe any midwifery applicant would write this badly. If you've got to the stage of applying for jobs, you certainly know how to work in a team and provide excellent midwifery care which keeps clients safe. However, let's think about why this application isn't a good one.

Where this application went wrong. It showed:

1. Poor skills around communication to coordinators and other team members, and alarming practice around managing obstetric emergencies, a very concerning attitude for any midwife but particularly a newly qualified member of staff who will need to know when to ask for help in order to keep clients safe.
2. A lack of insight and interest in diversity, concerning practice around language barriers and individualized care.
3. Poor prioritization skills, and lack of insight into audit or clinical governance.
4. Some interest in being a practice supervisor but a lack of understanding of the need for delegation and professional responsibility.
5. A lack of advocacy skills, possible issues with informed choice and consent around students and 'making use of birth'; also a very concerning lack of reporting of poor care regarding women feeling 'belittled'.

6. A lack of empathy for the staff members; remember that blame culture can be a cause of unsafe care.

7. Some mention of wanting to develop skills as a qualified midwife would be fine but talking about a lack of expertise with CTG traces is a problem. CTGs can be tricky but are ultimately something newly qualified midwives should have some expertise with, as a limited skills in this area could be very dangerous.

Now let's take a look at a strong personal statement.

A well-written personal statement

Box 10.2: A longer personal statement – good technique

During my training I have given high-quality care while supported by qualified staff. My training took place primarily in antenatal, labour and postnatal wards, as well as community settings, and I also gained experience in the High Dependency Unit, Fetal Medicine Clinic and specialist midwifery teams including the Rainbow Team for vulnerable clients, the Homebirth Team, and Safety and Governance.

My practice has included facilitating 25 midwifery-led healthy straightforward births in the Danebury Birth Centre, and much of this care also included breastfeeding support in line with UNICEF baby friendly guidelines. The Birth Centre is able to facilitate a 40% waterbirth rate, and I feel lucky to have gained so much experience with these kinds of births and also uncomplex care in general. This will help me in being a lead professional in universal midwifery care settings.

I have also gained experience in additional care need areas. These have ranged from monitoring hypertension and PET, SGA and IUGR screening, intrapartum care including induction of labour with prostaglandins and/or syntocinon, CTG interpretation, managing both elective and emergency caesarean births and instrumental deliveries, as well as emergencies including bradycardia and postpartum haemorrhage. The obstetric and neonatal medical teams have been informative and supportive as we communicated together to ensure sound decision making during complex care. I have an awareness of the A-EQUIP model of supervision, and have accessed PMA support after complex care that was fast-moving, which was helpful in learning from situations that were particularly well managed by the multidisciplinary team. My training has also included comprehensive learning to ensure I can document to the required standard using patient care software and I have experience of incident forms and when we use them. I have been able to work with highly experienced midwives and benefit from their comprehensive knowledge and I have also gained the ability to work under pressure and manage my time well. In total, I have trained for over 2,300 hours, in varied shift patterns, including on-call, and would plan to offer this flexibility as a qualified member of staff.

Working with junior students has been a particularly rewarding area for me, and I enjoy seeing each individual's confidence grow as they gain new skills. This has also been good practice for me in terms of how much to delegate and how much to directly oversee and has given me empathy for and understanding of the role of practice supervisors. I look forward to upskilling in this area. I also have experience with skills needed for a band 6 role including catheterization, venepuncture, cannulation and collecting blood cultures, as well as health promotion roles like discussing vaccinations. I intend to have a proactive attitude and continue to gain skills upon qualification so I can work towards further autonomy, which will be satisfying for me but also of benefit to clients who will gain more continuity in their care.

I have enjoyed working in a multicultural trust and have an awareness of how to facilitate the needs of women, pregnant people and their families, around religious, spiritual or other personal needs. I am aware of MBRRACE findings around Black and brown clients facing far greater risks during childbearing and have been inspired in my practice to be extra vigilant, and also keep up to date with all efforts in this area.

My dissertation was on the screening tools used to pick up on Small for Gestational Age or Growth Restricted babies, the level of evidence we use in choosing intervention and how to support clients in their choices. I was encouraged to send this piece of work to MIDIRS Midwifery Digest and it is being considered for publication. Along with Saving Babies Lives and Each Baby Counts initiatives, trust guidelines have been important in showing me how applying research evidence can help result in reducing poor outcomes. I find this fascinating and heartening, and also place great value on offering individualized support and information for each client, so they can make a care plan in partnership with their midwives and the multi-professional team. This is the outlook I bring with me to become a newly qualified midwife and I have aspirations to one day work in fetal medicine.

In the summer of 2019, I volunteered with the Yoga Babies company, who offer gentle but strengthening exercise and relaxation classes during pregnancy and the postnatal period. Through this, I refreshed my physiology knowledge and I also gained skills around the use of breath work in anxiety-provoking or painful situations. There was also a big social element in these groups. I used my active listening skills and was rewarded by forming relationships with women (some of who have recognized me and approached me in practice). It was a privilege to understand experiences and to see clients' confidence and well-being grow. My own yoga practice has helped me with work/life balance and well-being throughout my training and will continue to support me as a newly qualified midwife.

I look forward to working through band 6 proficiencies and working as a qualified competent midwife for many years to come.

What this statement did well

This statement was written well, with good spelling and grammar, which helps to show excellent communication skills. A warm, empathetic manner also comes through. It also showed the following.

1. Excellent respect for and collaboration with both junior and experienced staff, and experience of and ability in obstetric emergency situations.

2. An understanding of the different specialists that work together in perinatal care, including safeguarding and bereavement teams.

3. Experience of normal birth, breastfeeding and waterbirth, so overall a good grounding in key midwifery skills.

4. A wide range of experience in medical settings for midwifery clients with complex needs, and great time management and organizational skills to be able to follow this through.

5. Insight into documentation, audit and clinical governance.

6. Insight into the role of a qualified midwife in terms of delegation and beginning to supervise students.

7. An insight into advocacy and those at risk of inequitable care.

8. An impressive ability to link theory and academic ability to practice, as evidenced by a possible up-and-coming publication of a dissertation, and insight into current reports and care bundles.

9. Evidence of rapport-building skills and a true desire to work in partnership, based on voluntary work, and an indication of a good work/life balance and attitude to physical and emotional well-being.

Advice from midwives

If you're feeling stressed about starting to write your statement, have a look at the tips and tricks in Box 10.3 to get you started.

Box 10.3: Tips and tricks for starting personal statements

- Make a big mind map of all the relevant skills, experiences and insights you have gained throughout training. You may also want to include strengths you have gained in your personal life or your career before midwifery.

- Print the job description and specification documents and highlight the key skills, experiences and insights being asked for, and then build your statement around the most important ones.

- Start with simple ideas and build to more complex ones to achieve a piece of writing which flows.

- As a general rule, cover over one point, i.e. a skill, experience or insight, in about 150 words. However, adapt this as needed: easy-to-explain concepts like basic IT competency will need just a quick mention, whereas others like obstetric emergencies will need to cover more ground.

Box 10.4: Examples of key skills and experiences you may want to include in your statement

Time management

Providing health education for clients

Awareness of supervision, regulation and legal aspects of midwifery responsibilities

Normal childbearing, promotion of this

Breastfeeding/chestfeeding support

Managing complex care

Resuscitation, adult and neonatal and obstetric emergencies

Multidisciplinary teamwork

IT skills

Clinical skills like venepuncture, cannulation, suturing

Delegation, supervising junior members of the team

Meeting cultural needs of clients, valuing equality and diversity

Awareness of audit and risk management

Evidence-based care, interest in research

How to write your personal statement

Once you've identified what you need to include in your statement, you're ready to write up.

In your introduction or first sentence, explain what you have to offer the trust. Most people reading a piece of writing will pay attention to the first sentence more than any other part, so I would make the most of this prime real estate.

In terms of structure, the 'PEE' acronym stands for 'Point, Evidence, Explain' and is a good, simple way of setting out your skills. To make sure you're on target, you can also use the 'so what' rule when writing. For every sentence, ask 'so what?' as in 'Why should my prospective employer care? What does this do to allow them to offer me an interview?' To quote senior midwife Nabila Fowles-Gutierrez, 'when you're writing an application you need to use your emotional intelligence: think about the needs of the organization. Think about how best you can achieve their goal.'

Often you can achieve this best by showing rather than telling, so use examples. If the manager reading your statement can imagine you visually being a great midwife, almost like you've made a little film play in their head, it will make it easy for them to see why to hire you.

Another strong move is to refer to the trust values of where you want to work; most organizations will have a short phrase such as 'safe, caring, exceptional' to represent their aims, and you can discuss why these apply to your work as a midwife. You could also think about referring to current reports or care bundles, or perhaps government body guidance, policy documents or any legal responsibilities, for example, the NMC '4 Ps'. Part of a manager's role is to make crucial midwifery responsibilities clear to their staff, so anything like this will be music to their ears. Finally, you could add a work/life balance section to show a little about your personality, and how you plan to avoid burnout.

When you've finished writing, you could ask a friend, or even better, a qualified midwife friend, or your tutor at university, to read through for you and check for any additions that need to be made, as well as checking your spelling and grammar.

Shorter personal statements

I have also come across applications where your statement has to be no more than 300 words, which is quite the challenge. If this is the case, you will have to pare down and just include key themes.

Box 10.5: Example of a shorter personal statement

My training took place in all areas of this trust, and has covered universal care and complex care, as well as time with specialist teams. I see communication with midwifery colleagues and the multidisciplinary team to be the key factor in care, especially when there are fast-moving emergencies. I was pleased to gain experience in the midwife-led unit, which included waterbirth. My documentation skills have been praised and I have an understanding of clinical governance, audit and research, and the use of incident forms to improve care. I am passionate about the experiences of clients and would always aim to prioritize people, practise effectively, preserve safety and promote professionalism and trust. I have practised and learnt from midwives who are passionate about care being equally safe for all clients, especially those who are from ethnic minority backgrounds, or who have a constellation of medical needs (MBRRACE 2020). My dissertation focused on Small for Gestational Age babies and is being considered for publication by MIDIRS. I have a keen interest in reducing poor outcomes by using care bundles and evidence-based care. Each client has their own individual needs, and when we see them it is likely one of their most important moments, so I hold dignity, privacy and compassion as key values. I am interested in the outcomes improved by continuity of care and I would enjoy working in this model, as well as gaining more experience in skills such as suturing and cannulation within the hospital. Danebury is my home trust, where I had my children, and I look forward to working towards band 6 proficiencies and being a qualified competent midwife. In my spare time, I volunteer with 'Yoga Babies' and have my own yoga practice which helps with work/life balance.

Writing an application using a CV and cover letter

If you've been asked to submit a CV, your aim is to put together a summary document that makes your skills very simple for employers to understand. As you'll see, writing a CV and cover letter is very similar to a personal statement, it's just a slightly different layout, but all the essentials are the same.

Box 10.6: Example cover letter and CV

Name
Phone number
Email address
Home address

Professional Summary:

Student experience from 2 different trusts. Rotational experience across antenatal, intrapartum and postnatal care, and within specialist teams. Up-to-date obstetric emergencies training. In-depth knowledge from writing a dissertation on care bundles used nationally to reduce poor outcomes. Excellent time management skills and commitment to kind, compassionate care which respects the choices of women and pregnant people. Special interest in waterbirth.

Career Objectives:

To be a kind, caring, highly competent midwife working at Danebury Trust, moving to a band 6 position within the next year, and perhaps pursuing an interest in fetal medicine as a further goal.

Core Qualifications:

First class midwifery degree and NMC registration to be gained September 2019.

Excellent interpersonal skills based on developing relationships with midwifery clients over last three years on placement in all midwifery areas of Danebury Trust.

Experience:

I have involvement in the following situations and settings:

- Three years training, antenatal, intrapartum, postnatal care in hospital wards, community settings and including birth at home, in all shift patterns and with on-call components.

- Clinical skills including palpation, fundal height measurement, vaginal examination, venepuncture, catheterization and some experience with skills like cannulation and suturing.

- Caring for clients with complex care needs like pre-eclampsia, diabetes, epilepsy and for those with multiple pregnancies.

- Facilitating choices outside the guidelines, with skilled practice supervisor and consultant support.

- Continuity of care, which involved specialist teams in High Dependency Unit, Scan clinic, with vulnerable women's team.

- Incident reports and audit.

- Obstetric emergencies, taking more of a lead role during PPH and initiating first measures during shoulder dystocia and neonatal resuscitation, and experience as a member of the multidisciplinary team during complex neonatal resuscitation, bradycardia, cord prolapse and severe pre-eclampsia.

- Leading care during normal straightforward birth, including waterbirth.

- Supporting establishing breastfeeding, and assisting with challenges around supply, latch and positioning, and referring on, all in line with Unicef guidelines.

- Promotion of health for midwifery clients, including working with outside agencies that provide psychological support, addiction support such as stop smoking services and awareness of local parenting charities.

- Knowledge of IT systems and how to contemporaneously document care.

- Understanding of AEQUIP, supervision, clinical governance and trust values.

- Experience supporting junior students, with an interest in being a practice supervisor.

- Enjoyment of working with and providing for the needs of a multicultural and diverse client base, including LGBTQ+ needs.

- An interest in audit and research taking place in trusts, particularly the Danebury based FGR study.

Additional Employment Experience:

Healthcare Assistant: 2016–present

Clinical care including taking observations, fluid balance, personal care, cannula and catheter care. Bed changes and restocking. Building kind and compassionate relationships with clients. Reporting back to registered staff members. Wards included ICU, Neuro, Cardiac and Gynae.

Gym Receptionist at Nuffield Health: Nov 2013–Nov 2016

Excellent customer service in person, and phone etiquette.

Payment processing, subscriptions and computer systems experience.

Working independently and under pressure.

Additional Information:

- Member of midwifery society, involvement in organizing study day on bereavement

- Member of university climbing club

- Keen runner

Box 10.7: Midwifery cover letter

Dear Danebury Trust,

I am writing to you to apply for a band 5 midwife position working in a preceptorship role. I have experience in a neighbouring trust in all areas of antenatal, labour and postnatal care, at a stand-alone midwifery birth centre, and in the community. I have also been lucky to work in ICU as a healthcare assistant, and on one occasion as a senior student midwife following through with an ill patient with complex needs. I have worked in every type of shift and could offer flexibility and commitment as a qualified member of staff.

I have passion for normal birth, and have enjoyed personally facilitating five water births as part of my training. I also have an appreciation of complex care when women and pregnant people need multidisciplinary team. I understand the trust values are to be patient-centred, fair, collaborative, accountable and empowered and I am similarly minded.

I have had the opportunity to practise health promotion through conducting antenatal classes at my current trust and I find helping parents make the right choices for them to be very rewarding. I am aware of A-EQUIP as a supervision model and have accessed PMA support, for instance while advocating for the needs of a transgender client to make sure language choice and aims were clear to all staff before they attended scan clinic or the birth centre. I also enjoy breastfeeding/chestfeeding support and have shadowed a lactation consultant. I have experience with obstetric emergencies and for example have taken a lead role in the management of a PPH. I am up to date with 'Prompt' obstetric skills drills and adult and neonatal resuscitation days. I have been praised for contemporaneous documentation and I quickly understand new IT systems. I have begun to gain experience in new areas such as cannulation and suturing and look forward to developing these skills during the preceptorship period. I have been involved in recording information for audit, I have read the Danebury studies around fetal growth restriction and find the concept of early screening predicting the likelihood of early delivery to be fascinating. I would potentially like to work in fetal medicine one day.

Danebury care has a great reputation with both clients and staff and it would be an honour to complete my preceptorship, develop as a band 6 midwife and grow further into this profession within your trust.

Kind regards

Writing under pressure

Sometimes you might see an advert late and you have to write an application in a couple of hours. It might feel like you're not in with a chance but plenty of midwives get jobs under these circumstances. If this happens to you, keep it short, and perhaps skip describing previous employment if your experiences don't relate specifically to midwifery. I think these applications can come off really well sometimes, the writing can be fast-moving and full of enthusiasm.

Writing an application for a specialist role

I can't advise on applications for more specialist roles but I can suggest basic strategies like spending time reading journals and expert blogs, and perhaps getting a textbook on the subject. You could look at YouTube or Vimeo videos, and perhaps attend a conference or try to find conference transcripts (sometimes you can email the organizers of the conference and get hold of these). It would also be good to shadow someone in your specialist role; if this is not possible in your trust, because it might be unfair from an interview point of view, then ask a neighbouring trust if they have someone in a similar position you could talk to. Try to develop an idea of the priorities of the role and then find experiences in your own background that illustrate you can meet the requirements. Even if you're rejected, the worst that will happen is you spend a long time with the field you're interested in, which is excellent preparation for a future interview.

If you're going for something really competitive, you might even want to consider writing an article or review on that particular area. Journals like The Practising Midwife or MIDIRS are always looking for high-quality content. If you're struggling for journal access, try and look for your nearest medical library or university that has healthcare students and ask if you can come in to use their computers.

One other thing I thought was very interesting is when senior midwife Kelly Williams, who is lead midwife for the NHS North Thames Genomic Medicine Service, commented that 'One of the things you need to know is that a job specification is an employer's wish list. It's not a must-have list. I am especially aware of this having been in the position of hiring people.' Assume you have what it takes and build from there.

Kelly also told me about her involvement in the Florence Nightingale Windrush Foundation. This is a Health Education England Programme that offers nurses and midwives who are descendants of the Windrush generation or are from ethnic minority backgrounds support with their career development (Williams 2021). If you are Black or brown, I might suggest reading Kelly's interview on midwifediaries.com.

In the appendix to this book there is a list of interviews with midwives in specialist roles which feature on midwifediaries.com, so perhaps check this out for help in specific areas.

Interviews

Very few of our life paths depend entirely on the outcome of a single interview, though I know it can feel that way. You might want to look at the section on nerves in Chapter Three and the suggestions about interpersonal dynamics in Chapter Nine. Aim for a calm demeanour, and remember that the staff interviewing you are looking for safety and potential, not perfection. It also might be helpful to know that newly qualified midwives report that these interviews tend to be positive experiences. Interviewers will know you are newly qualified and likely to be nervous, and they will want you to do well.

> My interview was lovely because the interviewers were so nice and tried really hard to make me feel relaxed. I felt as prepared as you can feel, but I doubt anyone goes in feeling fully prepared. I think it's important to

remember they are rooting for you! It's helpful to ask mentors for advice and to brush up on some hot topics. The hardest part was overcoming nerves and trying to articulate things. Remember that you are also screening them as a potential employer so if you aren't getting good vibes then maybe you wouldn't want to work there?

Em Gibson

I think this is great advice.

You might also want to spend a bit of time getting into the interviewer's shoes. What are they looking for? What would be the best outcome for them? Probably they want to hire a brilliant, safe junior midwife who will go on to do great things for the trust. What would be the worst outcome? For them to miss some indication that you will be unsafe. So your interviewer will be on the lookout for midwives who can function safely in a variety of situations, including emergencies, and they will also be looking for passion and drive. In addition, you could talk about your ambitions, because we need more midwifery leaders and midwives who want to make a difference in specialist fields.

Using the same kind of language that you would use in clinical practice, for instance 'early warning sign', 'care plan', 'obstetric review', etc., is a good idea as it will help the interviewers to imagine you in practice. An interview is probably not the place to discuss failings of the trust you're training with, or failings of your university, as this is complex territory which will require a lot of explanation and is not about your skills. However, you could talk about clinical governance, and how trusts achieve high quality of care. You could also talk about current models of supervision; for instance, the A-EQUIP model in the UK, which amongst other things tries to support midwives in solving their challenges autonomously. You could also talk about some of the key documents midwives should be aware of; in the UK at the time of writing this might be the Ockenden report and MBRRACE. However, some new midwives who have not been successful in being offered a job after their first interview have sometimes reported feedback that they gave answers that were complex or that they analysed policies in detail, but didn't cover the basics well enough. Remember that this is an interview to check you will be an asset to the team at a band 5 level, rather than being for a Master's programme or specialist role. You can of course go into as much detail as you find interesting, but only if you have first shown you can be an excellent clinical team member.

Before you go into your interview, have any identification documents ready and have your phone turned off. If you're doing a remote interview, check your video feed with a friend beforehand and make sure you have a professional background. It's hard to give proper eye contact during a remote interview but I find looking into the camera every so often can help replicate this.

Dress smartly, as you would for any interview. The trust or organization might ask you to come dressed in uniform which could make things more simple. I would revise the trust values so you can incorporate these in at least one answer.

If you are attending in person, take your portfolio; it will likely be ready as a component of your course but if not you can revisit the Presentations chapter. Include particularly good grades, some reflections which show your best care and thank you cards which have been anonymized. These can all help make a great impression.

Interview questions

It's worth asking practice supervisors at your hospital or workplace if there is a trust 'question bank' that you can have a look at. Or just ask what the interviews are like. You can always say 'don't give me an unfair advantage or anything, but do you have any advice ... '; it's a good idea to see what support or information is available to you.

Otherwise, you can make a list of the questions that you think are most likely to come up and then look at the relevant topic areas. You can also use the 'What question would I be most unhappy about coming up?' strategy to help with your revision.

Another strategy that works well but that hardly anyone takes the time to do is recording yourself on camera to see what you look like interviewing. Often there are small changes to your phrasing or body language that you can make that will help the interviewers see your confidence and what you'll be like in practice. For instance, check you're not frowning or touching your face and hair too much, try to have the same attitude that you bring to caring for clients.

Have a go with the sample interview questions below.

Initial questions:

- Why would you like to be a midwife at our trust?
- Tell us about your training.
- Have you done any extended projects or other roles that could help you as a midwife?
- What has been the most challenging thing about training?
- Where do you see yourself in five years' time?

Scenario questions:

- You're working on a ward and one of your midwifery clients has been discharged and is just about ready to go home. You hear her buzzer, go into her side room, and see she appears to be unconscious on the bed. You can see some blood pooling underneath her. Tell me what you'd do next.
- You're working in recovery and note a baby has a temperature of 36.4 degrees centigrade. Tell me what you'd do next.
- You are doing a postnatal visit on day 5, and note the baby has lost 11 per cent of their birth weight. The baby is breastfed and all other elements of your checks and their history indicate things are normal. Tell us about the care plan you might have.
- You're the first midwife to arrive at a home birth. You have found that the client is in established labour. Tell us about the care plan you might have.

Questions about being a qualified midwife:

- What do you know about revalidation?
- Tell me about any important national documents you've read about and how this has informed your practice
- Should we ever apologize to midwifery clients?
- What are your personal qualities and experience that will contribute to good midwifery care in the trust?
- Tell us about how you might manage a day you're not enjoying at work.
- What would you do if you had concerns about a client's care and the doctor you were contacting was not concerned?

You will probably have an opportunity to ask questions at the end of the interview. Sometimes our anxiety can bubble over and we can ask questions like 'How many positions are you making available for newly qualified staff?'

Remember that asking a question is another opportunity to show your strengths, so something like 'What kind of breastfeeding training does your trust provide?' or 'What kind of support is in place for staff to transition to band 6?' might be more positive.

Further strategies

Revising obstetric emergencies, such as adult resuscitation, neonatal resuscitation, bradycardia, pre-eclampsia and eclamptic seizure, sepsis, shoulder dystocia and cord prolapse is a good idea. You should be able to use the same resources as for your final year OSCEs.

Identify the situation you're being asked about, so say aloud 'PPH' or 'shoulder dystocia', etc., so your interviewer can follow your thoughts. Remember your SOAPS, i.e. call for help using the emergency buzzer and ask for a senior midwife, obstetrician, anaesthetist and paediatrician as needed. Start the basics of care. So for a PPH this might be asking for the PPH trolley, giving syntocinon, delivering the placenta, getting cannulas in and starting fluids, catheterizing, taking blood and so on. You probably don't need to talk about every drug and every dose, or the physiology behind each manoeuvre, though if you can, great. Remember to think about any drugs or procedures that are a doctor's responsibility and whether they are the best person to take charge of care. After you've reached the end of the emergency, think about documentation, supporting the midwifery client and their family and any follow-up care you can think of. Privacy and dignity are always components of good midwifery care.

Some interviews include group work in emergency situations. Most applicants strategize for these by pretending they really are in that practice situation. Group work can be challenging if you don't know each other but everyone will be feeling the same. Act as sensibly and safely as you can and you'll be doing a great job.

Multiple mini interview questions

This is a slightly different kind of interview.

MMIs were developed within the last fifteen years and started in an American medical school. The school noticed that standard one-to-one interviews didn't predict how well doctors performed when they started training. They were concerned that vital skills like empathy, compassion, interpersonal ability and ethical reasoning were not assessed well enough in standard interviews. MMIs were created as a way of assessing prospective medical student's skills more accurately. This style of interview is now used to choose students for other healthcare courses, and for hiring clinicians in the UK and other countries.

Different interviewers will score your answers. When these interviews have been run in person, interviewees have moved between different interview stations. The idea is you are appraised by many different interviewers who do not share their impressions with each other, which should mean a fairer assessment (Astroff 2022).

Especially during Covid, interviews have been remote which means you're more likely to be given a series of questions by just a couple of interviewers working together but the basic concept remains the same.

Multiple mini interviews usually concentrate on scenarios and though you may have some like the ones listed above that are based on emergencies, they might be more unusual.

For instance:

> You are working on a busy antenatal ward. You have various patients needing care: one patient is having her labour induced and is asking for pain relief; one patient needs blood taking for pre-eclampsia (PET); one patient needs admitting for induction; and one patient who is annoyed and wants to know if they can go for a cigarette despite being on IV antibiotics. You have a maternity care assistant working with you. How would you organize your time?

In answering this kind of question you should think about:

- Empathy, compassion, emotional intelligence, the ability to offer dignity and respect
- Ability to reflect, learn and improve
- Ability to advocate
- Safety and clinical excellence in midwifery situations
- Ability to work well with the multidisciplinary team
- Knowing when and who to ask for help
- Excellent documentation

Remember that everyone is in the same boat. When I don't know where to start in answering a question, I'll often go back to my standard midwifery answer structure:

- Common sense
- Midwifery responsibilities
- Social and ethical considerations
- Who's most vulnerable and have you controlled for this?

Box 10.8: Sample MMI answer

Common sense

Overall, a patient being induced and wanting pain relief could possibly be progressing, so it's important to prioritize their care.

I would ask my maternity assistant colleague to go and see the patient who is annoyed and wants to go for a cigarette. They would need to explain that I will be there as soon as I can but as only registered staff members can stop IV infusions, and I am busy caring for other patients, they may have to wait. Perhaps the maternity care assistant could then go to the patient waiting to be admitted, or depending on the practice area, a ward clerk might be able to show this patient to their bed and buzzer.

The PET bloods could possibly be taken by a competent student or care assistant but that would be something I could get to a bit later if these options weren't possible.

Midwifery responsibilities

My responsibilities would lie with the patient in immediate need of midwifery care. Since I am the registered staff member the responsibility lies with me. This means I would want to go to the patient who is most likely to be in active labour and work out whether they need transferring for one to one care. Pain relief is also a human right so I would want to prioritize their care for this reason as well.

Social and ethical considerations

It is important the patient who wants a cigarette has the correct support. We offer stop smoking help but smoking is still a personal choice and it must be frustrating to have to ask to go out. Sometimes a patient uses the excuse of smoking to simply have a break from the ward and it's important to support well-being. If the patient is too ill to go out we could offer some nicotine gum. Hopefully, we will be able to ask the patient if they can stay on the ward until the IV antibiotics are finished, otherwise it becomes a complicated task as we will need to stop and start the infusion and work out timings accordingly. This patient might need compassionate listening time from staff and it's worth checking if they have been offered stop smoking help as well, though possibly not while they are feeling frustrated.

It's a better situation to be in if every patient can be admitted, given a tour and shown their buzzer on arrival. Induction can be a daunting process and everyone deserves a warm welcome and to know who is looking after them. I'd hope I could get to them as soon as possible and check they've made an informed choice in terms of induction.

I also wouldn't want to neglect the patient with PET; hopefully they've been told to press their buzzer if they have any symptoms like a headache, visual disturbance, stiff neck, nausea or vomiting, epigastric pain or oedema, or any concerns about fetal movements.

Who's most vulnerable and have you controlled for this

Overall I would hope the ward was well staffed enough for patient buzzers to be answered and no one to be neglected. When it's busy you all need to work as a team. Every patient is admitted to an antenatal ward for a reason, and while my immediate attention would be the client who needs pain relief and possibly more clinical support, everyone's needs are important. If there were not enough staff I might bleep the duty manager to get help. If no help was available it would be important to put in an incident form about staffing.

To conclude

The experience of job hunting as a newly qualified midwife varies widely. Some trusts will hire all the new midwives finishing their training without even interviewing. In other areas, there are only a couple of positions and that's a really difficult situation to be in as you'll be competing with your student colleagues. The good news is that as a qualified midwife, you will never be short of a job if you can move; the bad news is that getting a job might mean moving location for a while to build up your skills.

Be enthusiastic, professional and leave the staff interviewing you in no doubt that you would love to work in that specific trust, especially if the position you want has a lot of competition. If you happen to be rejected, remember that this has nothing to do with your ability and does not predict the outcome of any other interview. Getting into much-sought-after midwifery roles depends on being the right person at the right time, and persistence if it doesn't work out to begin with.

It's worth remembering that your first interview for a qualified midwife role is a proud moment for everyone, you've nearly made it. It's likely that the staff interviewing you will be cheering you on.

Being a Newly Qualified Midwife

11

Introduction

In this final chapter we'll think about working as a newly qualified midwife – you made it! We'll cover your first shifts, time management and prioritization from a qualified point of view, and the skills you'll need to work through as part of your newly qualified period, often known as 'preceptorship'. We'll also talk about a few practical matters, like how best to receive constructive criticism, and getting used to delegation. Finally, we'll discuss the emotional side of the transition.

Your first shifts as a qualified midwife

Everyone is nervous on their first shift working as a newly qualified midwife. It's a different feeling from being a student as you are now legally accountable for the care you're giving. However, supporting newly qualified midwives is a common occurrence in any maternity hospital or community setting, and coordinators and other members of staff will be aware that you're just starting out. To quote labour ward coordinator and midwifery lecturer Carinna Griffiths, 'the net under you that was there as a student doesn't just disappear' (2021).

Time management and prioritization

Time management and prioritization were the hardest-won skills for me. The golden rule is not to compare yourself to anyone else around you as you're not slow, you're just newly qualified. Being a midwife is an enormous role, and experienced staff may well have forgotten how long it took them to get fast.

You should have supernumerary time so you can work alongside another midwife for your first few shifts, and it's great if this is with your 'preceptor' member of staff who has been assigned to help you through your newly qualified period. However, service pressures sometimes mean you end up being autonomous straight away. If you're in this situation, identify the nearest friendly midwife and periodically check in with them. Asking a supportive midwife to double check your care plan is actually a good policy for well into your preceptorship period, if not your whole career.

Preceptorship sign-off books and other requirements

The next goal you're likely to have is passing your preceptorship period. In the UK this means transitioning from band 5 to band 6. Most trusts will have a programme with skills to get signed off, and some will require you to have worked a certain number of hours before you can do this.

When I was newly qualified, having a clear idea of the kind of skills expected of me was useful in helping me feel I was progressing and doing a good job. Just like with undergraduate placement sign-off books, preceptorship sign-off books can be a little hard to navigate, probably because requirements change frequently.

You might want to use Trello or another management app for this kind of task as you will be able to easily access your notes on a computer or phone. It's worth pointing out that lots of midwives just get on with it, and this works fine, but I get a lot of energy from being organized in this way, so I'll share the information in case you're a nerd like me.

Box 11.1: Preceptor competency checklist

Books to complete

- Medications
- Blood Transfusion Pack
- Blood Gas Analyser Pack
- IV Drugs

Guidelines to read

- Bereavement Policy
- Patient Group Directions Policy
- Oxygen Administration
- Anti-D Guideline

Skills to demonstrate under supervision

- Cannulas sited under supervision (5)

Meetings with preceptor

- Initial
- 3-month review

Questions to ask practice development team

- How to complete single-handed drug administration
- How to complete antenatal and postnatal checklists

Study days

- Breastfeeding Study Day booked
- Breastfeeding Study Day attended
- Infection Control Study Day booked
- Infection Control Study Day attended
- Neonatal Study Day booked
- Neonatal Study Day attended

Your A–Z book

You may still have your student A–Z book will contain phone numbers, IT tips and other bits of information. Or if you're moving trusts, you may want to start a new one. You can also buy 'lot to remember' midwifery cards or, as I mentioned in a previous chapter, you can buy transparent ID card holders made of soft plastic, which are perfect for reminders that you can keep on your lanyard. For example, you might want easy reference versions of CTG classifications, observation protocols, fontanelles and sutures for the identification of position during vaginal examinations and so on.

It is worth pointing out that you are not supposed to know all the guidelines yet. A practice development midwife once told me she found newly qualified midwives don't want to be seen looking up guidelines because it shows their lack of experience. In reality, it's actually reassuring to see newly qualified midwives doing this and if anyone asks about it you can say 'getting things correct is really important to me, I like to double check'.

You could also keep a list of things you've done well in the front of your A–Z book, which will help you remember your strengths.

Delegating

Delegating can feel weird, especially if the Maternity Care Assistant or whoever else you're working with is more experienced/older than you. Remember that you're all working together so if you're asking them to do tasks, they are equal to you but with a different scope of practice. If it still feels weird, ask yourself if you want a Care Assistant to do a job because you don't want to do it, or because you're too busy. If you're too busy and you're asking for help, that's effective delegation. Maternity Care Assistants will be able to do tasks like make beds, fetch water and meals for patients/clients, find equipment and restock, and take observations and report back if they are abnormal. You will also get experienced Maternity Care Assistants who can troubleshoot breastfeeding/chestfeeding issues, take blood and cannulate, and be a second at birth. To begin with, Maternity Care Assistants made sure I was a safe midwife, and I believe that's exactly how we should set things up; the least experienced staff should benefit from the most experienced, even across job roles. You can also watch experienced midwives and see what they do when they delegate; one of the best senior midwives I know is direct when asking people to do things, but always says thank you when she notices a task is complete. If you can remember the names of the staff members you're working with, this is a great idea and will get you a long way. Ward Clerks can help you with admissions, anything paperwork related, they tend to know where all the phone numbers are, they can request notes, admit patients, etc. You'll also find the more experienced Ward Clerks function as key members of the team. They will sometimes help you with safety concerns; for instance if they hear you saying 'I'm a bit worried about the person I'm looking after in room x, but none of the doctors are answering their bleeps' they may direct you towards a consultant number or another doctor covering the area who's likely to pick up.

The SBAR tool

Remember the SBAR tool? It's worth having another look at it from a qualified point of view. Using the SBAR tool to organize your notes for the shift can be useful for remembering when to ask for help. You could write 'Situation Background Assessment Recommendation' at the top of your handover sheet. Midwifery gets complicated and coming back to these basic principles will help you remember to do things.

So for example, if you're on a labour ward, you will probably have the following basics either on the sheet that's been printed for your shift or you can copy them off the whiteboard:

Zetty Eizak – G1P0 36+2 TPTL SROM cl liq 1100 GDM

I learnt an onboarding proforma from an obstetrics textbook that goes something like the following.

Box 11.2: Proforma summary for midwifery client

G

P

Gest

Hb

Blood type

Allergies

Med hx

Obstetric hx

Current:*

(* Current is where I'll note medications given, and I'll start to make a tick list of medications and observations, scans and anything else due at a particular time that shift.)

So if I were looking after Zetty, my sheet might look like the following.

Box 11.3: Handover sheet for 1:1 care of patient Zetty Eizak

G1

P0

Gest: 36+2

HB: 109

Blood type: A pos

Allergies: NKA

Med hx: nil of note

Obstetric hx: Scans NAD placenta anterior and clear of os. SROM 11am clear liquor 19/8/21, contractions intermittent since, GDM diet controlled

S: Ongoing cx 2:10

B: As above, SROM yesterday, TPTL

A: CTG ongoing, has not met Dawes Redman criteria as lack of accelerations, reduced variability for 40 minutes

R: For position change to left lateral and encourage to drink clear fluids, if CTG does not meet criteria by 50 minutes for obstetric review and to consider conservative methods, cannula and IV fluids. Have let shift leader know.

Especially if it's busy, I might think the SBAR bit through instead of writing it out. But even if this is the case, I still try to write down the 'recommendation' part as this is the most important element of the SBAR, and one that can be forgotten when you're new. Keep asking yourself, 'Am I fulfilling my advocacy role? Am I keeping things safe?' In this case, have you implemented your plan with the position change and fluids, and let a senior staff member know what's going on? In midwifery, situations can change quickly, don't let perfectionism be a 'twenty-ton shield' that gets in the way of you checking in with others (Brown 2012: 129).

Constructive criticism

In my first year of practice, I was unbelievably sensitive about criti-cism. The trick is to incorporate anything you think is useful back into your practice, and if you get the same feedback over and over, that probably means you have an area to work on. But just like in any profession that's busy and full of new relationships, you can let a lot of criticism go. In terms of self-criticism, it's probably a good idea to hold judgement on yourself until you're a year or so into being qualified, as you won't have the experience to give yourself a reasonable perspec-tive until then. Easier said than done, I know.

Reporting poor care

Hopefully, if you identify poor care in practice you will be able to speak to the professional in question there and then, as a 'firm, polite challenge is sometimes all that is needed' (Care Quality Commission 2021). If you can't do this, in the UK we have Professional Midwifery Advocates and Freedom to Speak up Guardians who you can talk to about anything concerning that you have witnessed, and I'm sure there are similar schemes wherever you are in the world. Incident forms are also routinely filled in for circumstances like care being delayed, important screening checks being missed or certain obstetric emergencies – see your trust policies for details. Incident forms can also be used to report issues like poor culture and you won't need to name individual members of staff. If you're still concerned or you think you need to whistle-blow, please see Chapter Nine for more help.

Breaks and holidays

In terms of managing time on shift, when I was first qualified, I would find myself skipping meal breaks so I could get everything done. This is a common reaction to the new level of responsibility. However, these days having a break is a priority for me, and even though often the clinical situation makes it impossible, when I can get a break I know this helps me with productivity, learning and avoiding mistakes.

One book for newly qualified midwives I've read suggests you shouldn't work full time for more than four months before taking a holiday or you'll be too tired to enjoy it (Agnew and Williams 2011). There's something to be said for resting before your holiday if you can, so you can make the most of the social and other healing stuff you'll get up to.

Celebrating and the emotions that come with the transition to newly qualified

The day I got signed off, I cried. I remember the midwife working with me was moved and I think my tutor was proud, though she was fairly inscrutable – it must be quite the responsibility to let midwives you've trained go off into the wild. I still had a few more shifts to go and things to get signed off. Like many big transitions, it felt like a series of small efforts joined together rather than one big cathartic moment.

I want to normalize the 'baby blues' that can come with being newly qualified. Big changes generally come with a mix of feelings. Make sure you do something to mark the occasion, like a special meal out or a night to celebrate with your cohort. There's usually some kind of graduation party. I did go to mine, and I love my cohort, we were a good group. But I'm not really one for big parties, so, instead, I ran a half marathon a month after qualifying and then went out for dinner. I think it was in the restaurant where it started to sink in.

Transitioning to being qualified is something that you will continually benefit from. Even if you decided to take a different kind of job and step away from being a midwife, no one can take away the fact that you passed the course and were on a professional register. It's like releasing your first album or publishing your first book: you've levelled up. But I don't think I began to breathe and enjoy things until the first waterbirth I provided solo care for, and that was six months into being a newly qualified midwife. I had been able to rest, and had enough money in the bank not to worry. It all felt okay.

To conclude

A common thought in the literature written to support newly qualified midwives, which also came up in a conversation I had with the lecturer/labour-ward coordinator I mentioned above, is that, to begin with, you might feel like you're not coping, and you may feel awkward about other members of staff stepping in to support you. But like in some corny montage from a film, when the next wave of newly qualified midwives turn up, you'll step in to help them and realize how far you've come (Griffiths 2021).

And then you realize, as with every achievement in life, the end of one goal is the beginning of another ...

Conclusion

They say we write the books we need. I'm going to miss this book so much. It's been my companion all the way through Covid, return to practice and getting to know the new hospital where I'm working. Bits of this book were very stressful to write but mostly it's just been a good thing to come back to.

When I was doing my A-Levels, I did Classical Civilisations, purely because I liked it and thought I'd never have the opportunity to study it again. In Classics, we read the Odyssey, and throughout it, Penelope, Odysseus' wife, is continually weaving a funeral shroud. She says she'll choose a new suitor when it's done. However, she unravels her weaving at the end of each day because she's loyal to Odysseus and even though by the end of the story he's been gone for twenty years, and everyone presumes him shipwrecked, she still believes he'll come home. Even in the years I took off from clinical practice, I was obsessed with midwifery and always hoped I'd return to it. With this book, I didn't purposely unravel anything at the end of each day but it's gone through a ton of iterative stages. I think it's been protective for me over this bumpy period of time. Even if your journey looks very different to mine, I hope the peer support is helpful and makes you experience the truth of training as a midwife, which is that no matter how alone you feel, there are midwives all over the world who right this second feel exactly like you.

Huge thanks to everyone who let me interview them; it's a career-affirming process. Each time I think our profession is stretched beyond anything we can handle, I find someone new who makes me feel hopeful and encouraged.

To end I want to reference the Master's capstone project written by May-Yen Flynn, one of the midwives whose full interview is on my website, midwifediaries.com.

At the end of her paper, she writes:

> I am reminded of how calm I feel in my role as an expert. A recent memory of a birth I assisted enters my mind. I remember glancing down at my Fitbit watch to memorise the timings of an imminent birth for my documentation later. The watch states that my pulse is 58 beats per minute, the same as when I am asleep. I notice that my body seems most relaxed while I am conducting a birth as I am comfortable suspended in this moment of uncertainty and unpredictability …

No matter how difficult midwifery feels while we are training and newly qualified, there's a level of expertise that will come with fluency. All the effort, every attempt, every failure counts. This is what we're aiming for.

Thanks for reading, much love, Eleanor (Ellie) Durant.

P.S. If you'd like to hear more from me, consider signing up to my mailing list on midwifediaries.com; much of my work is candid and focuses on emotional wellbeing.

Appendix
Your future career

In writing this book I conducted interviews with midwives who transitioned into specialist or other impressive roles within a few years of qualification. These are all super cool people, and many talked candidly about progressing their careers around significant adversity such as systemic racism, being the first person in their family to go to university or moving into a leadership role despite finding academic work to be a challenge. There's also one professional who found midwifery wasn't right for her and has built a different career using her experiences from the training.

I have quoted from many of these individuals in this book, but didn't have room to include their entire interviews. Instead, these can be found at midwifediaries.com. See below for their names and career paths.

Interview with Julia Reissmann, Perinatal Counselor

Interview with Charlie Day, Birth Trauma Resolution Practitioner

Interview with Nabila Fowles-Gutierrez, Public Health Researcher

Interview with Kelly Williams, Termination of Pregnancy Services Midwife, Manager, Researcher, Doctoral Student, and current Lead Midwife at North Thames Genomic Medicine Service Alliance

Interview with Carinna Griffiths, Midwifery Lecturer and Labour Ward Coordinator

Interview with Benash Nazmeen, Specialist Cultural Liason Midwife

Interview with Emma Bowles, Specialist Bereavement Midwife

Interview with Shannon McGill Randall, Infant Feeding Lead

Interview with May-Yen Flynn, Midwife and MSc Graduate

Bibliography

Abdaal, A. (2010) *The Power of Retrospective Revision Timetables*. aliabdaal.com

Abdaal, A. (2019) *How I Ranked 1st at Cambridge University – The Essay Memorisation Framework*. YouTube.

Abdaal, A. (2020) *How to Study for Exams – An Evidence-Based Masterclass*. Skillshare. skillshare.com/.

Agnew, C. and Williams, J. (2011) 'Now I am a Qualified Midwife', in J. Williams (ed.), *Midwifery Survival Guide: Common questions and answers for the newly qualified midwife*, 11. London: Quay.

Aldcroft, A. (2018) 'How to write and publish a paper'. *British Medical Journal (BMJ)*. https://bestpractice.bmj.com/info/wp-content/uploads/2018/12/How-to-write-and-publish-a-paper-2018.pdf.

Ali, S. (2021) 'Action to reduce maternal health inequalities'. BMJ Sexual & Reproductive Health blog. blogs.bmj.com/bmjsrh/.

All4Maternity (2020) 'In Conversation with Fatimah Mohamied'. Apple Podcasts.

Allen, D. (2015) *Getting Things Done: The art of stress-free productivity*. London: Piatkus Books.

Anderson, T. (2010) 'Researching Women's Views', in S. Wickham (ed.), *Appraising Research into Childbirth: An interactive workbook*, 44–64. Edinburgh: Elsevier Butterworth-Heinemann.

Andrews, R. (2007) 'Argumentation, critical thinking and the postgraduate dissertation'. *Educational Review*, 59 (1): 1–18.

Ashworth, E., Henchy, V. and McMahon, M. (2021) *Consent: rights in Childbirth*. AIMS [Workshop].

Association of Radical Midwives (ARM) (2017) *Albany Midwives Exonerated – ARM Demands Apology | Association of Radical Midwives*. midwifery.org.uk.

Astroff, R. (2022) 'History of the MMI'. [Interview].

Astrup, J. (2018) 'Blown off course'. *Midwives*, 21 (Winter): 36–40.

Barrass, R. (2005) *Students Must Write: A guide to better writing in coursework and examinations*. London: Routledge.

Birmingham City University (2019) *What to Wear on Placement*. bcu.ac.uk.

Birthrights (2017) *Birthrights Criticises NMC for Independent Midwives Decision*. birthrights.org.uk.

Birthrights (2019) *Human Rights in Maternity Care – Birthrights*. birthrights.org.uk.

Bloomfield, J., Pegram, A. and Jones, C. (2010) *How to Pass your OSCE: A guide to success in nursing and midwifery*. London: Routledge.

Bloomsbury (2019) *Cite Them Right Online*. citethemrightonline.com.

Bolton, G. and Delderfield, R. (2018) *Reflective Practice: Writing and professional development*, 5th edn. London: SAGE.

Breech Birth Network (2016) *About the Breech Birth Team*. Breech Birth Network. breechbirth.org.uk.

Brocklehurst, P., Hardy, P., Hollowell, J. et al. (2011) 'Perinatal and maternal outcomes by planned place of birth for healthy women with low-risk pregnancies: The birthplace in England national prospective cohort study'. *British Medical Journal*, 343.

Brown, A. (2019) *Informed is Best: How to spot fake news about your pregnancy, birth and baby*. London: Pinter & Martin.

Brown, B. (2010) *The Gifts of Imperfection*. Center City, MN: Hazelden.

Brown, B. (2012) *Daring Greatly: How the courage to be vulnerable transforms the way we live, love, parent, and lead*. London: Penguin Books.

Brown, B. (2021) *Atlas of the Heart: Mapping meaningful connection and the language of human experience*. London: Vermilion.

Brown, B. (2022) *Atlas of the Heart List of Emotions*. brenebrown.com.

Brown, P. (2014) *Make it Stick: The science of successful learning*. Cambridge, MA, and London: Harvard University Press.

Bryar, R. and Sinclair, M. (2011) *Theory for Midwifery Practice*. Basingstoke: Palgrave Macmillan.

Bryman, A. (2012) *Social Research Methods*. Oxford: Oxford University Press.

Bryson, B. (2019) *The Body: A guide for occupants*. New York: DoubleDay.

Burnett, A. (2021) 'Racism matters: this hurts us much more than it hurts you: the lived experiences of black, Asian and multi-racial student midwives'. *The Practising Midwife*, 24 (2). Also at All4Maternity. all4maternity.com.

Burney-Nicol, F. (2021) *The Lack of Black Midwifery Leadership at Board Level in the NHS in England –Why Aren't We Represented?* rcm. org.uk.

Cardiff University (2017) *Bachelor of Midwifery Preparation for Practice Placement Handbook*. Cardiff: HCARE, Cardiff University.

Care Quality Commission (CQC) (2021) *Raising a Concern with CQC*. cqc.org.uk.

Centers for Disease Control and Prevention (2019) *Racial and Ethnic Disparities Continue in Pregnancy-Related Deaths*. cdc.gov/.

Clarke, J. (2020) *How to Nail your Literature Review 1: Finding what you need*. Cambridge Researcher Development Programme, Cambridge University.

Cochrane Collaboration (2017) *Cochrane's 'logo review' Gets an Update*. community.cochrane.org.

Coomey, C. (2021) 'An exploration into why Black women are 5 times more likely to die in childbirth compared to White women'. Diss., Angela Ruskin University.

Cooper, S., Cant, R., Porter, J., et al. (2012) 'Simulation-based learning in midwifery education: a systematic review'. *Women and Birth*, 25 (2): 64–78.

Cronk, M. (2012) *Mary Cronk MBE: Her Renowned Famous Sayings*. Bernadette Bos. YouTube.

Cronk, M. and Graves, K. (2019) *Midwife Mary Cronk (MBE) Talks with Katharine Graves*. KGHypobirthing. YouTube.

Cunff, A. (2020) *How to Learn Anything with the Feynman Technique*. Ness Labs. nesslabs.com/.

Dahlgreen, W. and Shakespeare, A. (2015) *1 in 2 Young People Say They Are Not 100% Heterosexual*. yougov.co.uk.

Davis, M. (2013) *How to Assess Doctors and Health Professionals*. Chichester: John Wiley & Sons.

Delap, L. (2021) *Feminisms: A global history*. Milton Keynes: Pelican Books.

DMU (2022) *Decolonising DMU*. dmu.ac.uk.

Doyle, G. (2020) *Untamed*. New York: The Dial Press.

Drife, J. (2016) 'Fifty years of obstetrics and gynaecology'. *British Journal of Hospital Medicine*, 77 (Sup 10): 572–4.

Durant, E. (2014) *Student Midwife Fails*. YouTube.

Durant, E. (2015) *Should Midwives Have Tattoos? And Other Thoughts*. midwifediaries.com.

Durant, E. (2015a) *Midwife Uniforms: Professional or Opressional?* midwifediaries.com.

Edwards, N., Mander, R. and Murphy-Lawless, J. (2018) 'Introduction: A Toxic Culture', in N. Edwards, R. Mander and J. Murphy-Lawless (eds), *Untangling the Maternity Crisis*. London: Routledge, Taylor & Francis Group.

Ekechi, C. (2020) 'Christine Ekechi: How do we start a conversation about racism in medicine?' *British Medical Journal*, Blog (25 June). blogs.bmj.com/.

Elliott-Mainwaring, H. (2021) 'How do power and hierarchy influence staff safety in maternity services?'. *British Journal of Midwifery*, 29 (8): 430–9.

Ferriss, T. (2022) *80/20*. timferriss.com.

Fields, R. (2020) 'The brain learns in unexpected ways'. *Scientific American*, 1 March.

Foltz, B. (2020) *Statistics 101*. YouTube.

Gale Group (2008) *Viva Voce*. thefreedictionary.com.

Gibbs, G. (1998) *Learning by Doing: A guide to teaching and learning methods*. Oxford: Further Education Unit, Oxford Polytechnic.

Gibbs, G. (2010) *Graham R Gibbs*. YouTube.

Gilbert, E. (2015) *Big Magic*. New York: Penguin.

Gillen, P. (2021) *Bullying in Midwifery: Its Impact and How to Respond*. Maternity and Midwifery Forum. YouTube.

Gillen, P., Sinclair, M. and Kernohan, W. (2009) 'Student midwives' experience of bullying'. *Evidence Based Midwifery*, 7 (2): 46–53.

Godin, S. (2015) *Quieting the Lizard Brain*. YouTube.

Gould, J. (2017) 'Storytelling in midwifery: is it time to value our oral tradition?'. *British Journal of Midwifery*, 25 (1): 41–5.

Goyder, C. (2014) *Gravitas: Communicate with confidence, influence and authority*. London: Vermilion.

Greenhalgh, T. (2019) *How to Read a Paper: The basics of evidence-based medicine and healthcare*, 6th edn. Hoboken, NJ: John Wiley & Sons.

Greenwood, B., Hardeman, R., Huang, L. and Sojourner, A. (2020) 'Physician–patient racial concordance and disparities in birthing mortality for newborns.' *Proceedings of the National Academy of Sciences*, 117 (35).

Griffiths, C. (2021) Conversation with E. Durant [Interview].

Grobman, W., Rice, M., Reddy, U. M. et al. (2018) 'Labor induction versus expectant management in low-risk nulliparous women'. *New England Journal of Medicine*, 379 (6): 513–23.

Hale, J. (2019) *Five Things to Know about Being Disabled and LGBTQ*. open.edu.

Hargreaves, S. (2016) *Study Skills for Students with Dyslexia: Support for specific learning difficulties (SPLDS)*. Thousand Oaks, CA: SAGE Publications.

Hastie, C. (1996) 'Dying for the cause'. *Australian College of Midwives Incorporated Journal*, 9 (1).

Hatzigeorgiadis, A., Theodorakis, Y. and Zourbanos, N. (2004) 'Self-talk in the swimming pool: the effects of self-talk on thought content and performance on water-polo tasks'. *Journal of Applied Sport Psychology*, 16 (2): 138–50.

Heagerty, B. (1996) 'Reassessing the Guilty: The Midwives Act and the control of English midwives in the early 20th century', in M. Kirkham (ed.), *Supervision of Midwives*. Hale, Cheshire: Books For Midwives Press.

Health E-Learning and Media (2018) *OSCE Shoulder Dystocia Demonstration*. YouTube.

Heazell, A., Timms, K., Scott, R. et al. (2021) 'Associations between consumption of coffee and caffeinated soft drinks and late stillbirth—findings from the midland and north of England stillbirth case-control study'. *Obstetrical & Gynecological Survey*, 76 (6): 313–15.

Heylighen, F. and Vidal, C. (2008) 'Getting things done: the science behind stress-free productivity'. *Long Range Planning*: 21: 36–40.

Higher Education Staff Statistics (HESA) (2021) *Higher Education Staff Statistics: UK, 2020/21*. hesa.ac.uk.

Horner, J. (2021) Conversation with E. Durant [Interview].

Howes, V. and Muscat, H. (2015) 'Lethal fetal anomalies: a case of bilateral renal agenesis'. *MIDIRS Midwifery Digest*, 25 (3): 367–72.

Hughes, D. (2018) 'Midwifery lives matter'. *Midwifery Matters*, 156 (1).

Independent Maternity Review (2022) *Ockenden Report – Final: Findings, conclusions, and essential actions from the independent review of maternity services at the Shrewsbury and Telford Hospital NHS Trust* (HC 1219). London: HMSO.

Ingle, R. and Murphy-Lawless, J. (2019) 'Ireland's Midwives: "Stretched to beyond the point of breaking"'. The Women's Podcast: *The Irish Times*. [Podcast].

Jones, L. (2021) *Motivational Midwife*. YouTube.

Khan Academy (2016) *Mean, Median, & Mode Example*. [Video]. khanacademy.org.

Khan Academy (2018) *SQ3R: SAT active reading strategies (Part 1)*. khanacademy.org.

Khan Academy (2019) *Calculating Standard Deviation Step by Step*. khanacademy.org.

Kirkham, M. (1996) *Supervision of Midwives*. Hale, Cheshire: Books For Midwives Press.

Kirkham, M. (2007) *Traumatised midwives | AIMS*. aims.org.uk.

Knight, M., Bunch, K., Tuffnell, D. et al., eds. (2020) on behalf of MBRRACE-UK. *Saving Lives, Improving Mothers' Care – Lessons learned to inform maternity care from the UK and Ireland Confidential Enquiries into Maternal Deaths and Morbidity 2016–18*. MBRRACE.

Knight, M., Bunch, K., Tuffnell, D. et al., eds. (2021) *Saving Lives, Improving Mothers' Care – Lessons learned to inform maternity care from the UK and Ireland Confidential Enquiries into Maternal Deaths and Morbidity 2017–19*. MBRRACE.

Kunzler, A., Helmreich, I., Chmitorz, A. et al. (2020) 'Psychological interventions to foster resilience in healthcare professionals'. *Cochrane Database of Systematic Reviews* (5 July), 7 (7): CD012527.

Lord, M. (2022) 'abueladoula'. Instagram.

Lord, M. and Silver, A. (2021) *Allyship Webinar: Two leading lights in the birth world, specialising in racial inequalities and LGBTQ+ competency*. [Workshop].

Lundström, J., Mathe, A., Schaal, B. et al. (2013) 'Maternal status regulates cortical responses to the body odor of newborns'. *Frontiers in Psychology*, 4 (597).

MacLaren, I. (1984) *Be Kind: Everyone You Meet is Fighting a Hard Battle*. quoteinvestigator.com.

Mantle, R. (2020) *Higher Education Staff Statistics: UK, 2018/19 | HESA.* hesa.ac.uk.

Marques, E. (2021) 'The Data School – Pareto Chart – Don't Underestimate Your Peas'. thedataschool.co.uk.

Martin, G. (2019) *Statistics Made Easy!!! Learn about the t-test, the chi square test, the p value and more.* Global Health with Greg Martin. YouTube.

Massachusetts Institute of Technology (2014) *Confidence Intervals and Hypothesis Tests.* mit.edu.

McCool, M. (2009) *Writing around the World: A guide to writing across cultures.* New York: Continuum.

McGill-Randall, S. (2021) Conversation with E. Durant [Interview].

Medistudents (2017) *Top 10 Tips for Clinical Examinations.* medistudents.com.

Metcalf, H. and Hudson-Sharp, N. (2016) 'Inequality among lesbian, gay bisexual and transgender groups in the UK: a review of evidence'. Government Equalities Office. gov.uk.

Molloy, E., Biggerstaff, D. and Sidebotham, P. (2021) 'A phenomenological exploration of parenting after birth trauma: mothers' perceptions of the first year'. *Women and Birth*, 34 (3).

Montgomery v Lanarkshire Health Board [2015] (UKSC 11).

Moran, M. (2013) *Qualitative Sample Size.* statisticssolutions.com.

Mukwende, M., Tamony, P. and Turner, M. (2020) *Mind the Gap.* blackandbrownskin.co.uk/mindthegap.

Murphy-Lawless, J. (2014) *A Brief Glimpse into Hell.* aims.org.uk.

Murphy-Lawless, J. (2018) 'Responding to the tragedy of maternal death', in N. Edwards, R. Mander and J. Murphy-Lawless (eds), *Untangling the Maternity Crisis*, 133–41. London: Routledge, Taylor & Francis Group.

Nagoski, E. and Nagoski, A. (2019a) *Burnout.* London: Vermilion.

Nagoski, E. and Nagoski, A. (2019b) *Burnout* The XOXO Festival. YouTube.

Neiger, D. (2022) 'debsagos'. Instagram.

Newman, M. (2021a) Conversation with E. Durant [Interview].

Newman, M. (2021b) *Complications around childbirth: pre-eclampsia toxaemia (2014).* Via E. Durant. midwifediaries.com.

NHS (2017) *NHS England: ROAN Information Sheet 8: Confidentiality of Reflections for Appraisal*. england.nhs.uk.

NHS England (2017) *A-EQUIP: A Model of Clinical Midwifery Supervision A-EQUIP: An Acronym for Advocating for Education and Quality Improvement*. england.nhs.uk.

NMC (2020) *Ambitious for Change Research into NMC Processes and People's Protected Characteristics*. nmc.org.uk.

Oade, A. (2015) *Free Yourself from Workplace Bullying: Become bully-proof and regain control of your life*. Oxford: Mint Hall Publishing.

Oade, A. (2017) *Bullying in Teams: How to survive it and thrive*. Oxford: Oades Associates.

Office for National Statistics (2017) *Lesbian, Gay, and Bisexual People Say They Experience a Lower Quality of Life*. ons.gov.uk/.

Office for National Statistics (2021) *Sexual Orientation, UK: 2019*. ons.gov.uk/.

Ojanuga, D. (1993) 'The medical ethics of the "father of gynaecology"', Dr J Marion Sims'. *Journal of Medical Ethics*, 19 (1): 28–31.

Owens, D. and Fett, S. (2019) 'Black maternal and infant health: historical legacies of slavery'. *American Journal of Public Health*, 109 (10): 1342–5.

Papps, E. and Ramsden, I. (1996) 'Cultural safety in nursing: the New Zealand experience'. *International Journal for Quality in Health Care*, 8 (5): 491–7.

Patwari, R. (2015) *Odds Ratios and Risk Ratios*. YouTube.

Pendleton, J., Clews, C. and Cecile, A. (2022) 'The experiences of black, Asian and minority ethnic student midwives at a UK university'. *British Journal of Midwifery*, 30 (5).

Pennebaker, J. (1997) 'Writing about emotional experiences as a therapeutic process'. *Psychological Science*, 8 (3): 162–6.

Queen Mary University of London (2021) *People Profiles Series – Queen Mary University of London*. qmul.ac.uk.

Rankin, J. (2014) *Myles Midwifery A&P Colouring Workbook – E-Book*, 2nd edn. London: Churchill Livingstone.

RCM (2022a) *Government Undervaluing Midwifery Workforce is 'No joke', Says RCM*. rcm.org.uk.

RCM (2022b) *Position Statement: Safer Staffing Position Statement*. rcm.org.uk.

Reed, A. (2020) *Overdue: Birth, burnout and a blueprint for a better NHS*. London: Pinter & Martin.

Rees, C. (2011) *Introduction to Research for Midwives*, 3rd edn. London: Churchill Livingstone.

Reid, N. (2021) *The Good Ally*. London: Harper Collins.

Reissmann, J (2021) Conversation with E. Durant [Interview].

Reshr, E. and Tribole, E. (2020) *Intuitive Eating*. New York: St Martin's Essentials.

Richardson, S. (2020) *A Student Guide to Multiple Choice Exams*. uwec.edu.

Rolfe and Freshwater (2001) Critical *Reflection for Nursing and the Helping Professions: A User's Guide*, London: Red Globe Press.

Romiszewski, S. (2021) *Sleep Insomnia Expert UK*. sleepyheadclinic.co.uk.

Ryrie, A. (2015) *How We Learned that Slavery is Wrong*. Gresham College. YouTube.

Scanlan, S. and Walker, H. (2013) *Studying for Your Midwifery Degree*. SAGE: London.

Silver, A. J. (2017) *He's Not the Mother*. AIMS. aims.org.uk.

Silver, A. J. (2019) *Birth beyond the Binary*. aims.org.uk

Silver, A. J. (2021) Workshop. queerbirthclub.co.uk.

Simon Fraiser University (2013) *Exam Preparation: strategies for Open Book Exams | SFU Library*. lib.sfu.ca.

Spettel, S. and White, M. (2011) 'The portrayal of J. Marion Sims' controversial surgical legacy'. *The Journal of Urology*, 185 (6): 2424–7.

Sprouts (2017) *The Memory Palace: can you do it?* YouTube.

Squirrell, T. (2020) *How Many References Do You Need in an Essay?* timsquirrell.com.

Staffordshire University (2017) *Staffordshire University Poster Presentation Support for Student Midwives*. YouTube.

Stewart, M. (2010) 'Childbirth Interventions', in S. Wickham (ed.), *Appraising Research into Childbirth: An interactive workbook*, 77–8. Edinburgh: Elsevier Butterworth-Heinemann.

Stewart, S. (2020) 'Life and sarah-stewart'. blogspot.com.

Stillbirth and Neonatal Death Charity (SANDS) (2021) *14 to 13 Babies a Day – What's behind the Change?* sands.org.uk.

Sweet, L., Bass, J., Sidebotham, M., Fenwick, J. et al. (2019) 'Developing reflective capacities in midwifery students: enhancing learning through reflective writing'. *Women and Birth*, 32 (2): 119–26.

Tanabe, K. (2018) 'Pareto's 80/20 rule and the Gaussian distribution'. *Physica A: Statistical Mechanics and its Applications*, 510: 635–40.

The Royal College of Midwives (RCM) (2020) *First Five Years Forum (FFYF): Developing a preceptorship programme for newly qualified midwives in Scotland*. London: RCM.

The Undercover Midwife (2015) 'The undercover midwife: paracetamol and labour'. undercovermidwife.blogspot.com.

Turner, C., Farmer, J., Yousaf, H. et al. (2018) *Home | Civility Saves Lives | England*. civilitysaveslives.com.

Turner, F. (2018) *Be More Kind*. YouTube.

University College London (UCL) (2018) *Critical Reading Questions*. ucl.ac.uk.

University of Bangor (2021) *Using Visual Aids*. bangor.ac.uk.

University of Bath (2020) 'Understanding instruction words in academic essay titles'. blogs.bath.ac.uk.

University of Kent (2022) *Giving an Oral Presentation*. kent.ac.uk.

University of Leicester (2020) *Using Visual Aids*. https://studylib.net/doc/25390274/using-visual-aids.

Van der Riet, P., Rossiter, R., Kirby, D. et al. (2015) 'Piloting a stress management and mindfulness program for undergraduate nursing students: student feedback and lessons learned'. *Nurse Education Today*, 35 (1): 44–9.

Verghese, A. (2011) *A Doctor's Touch*. [Video] ted.com.

vnell12 (2012) *Cardiovascular Exam*. quizlet.com.

Von Kaisenberg, C. (2018) *The PROMPT Course Manual*. Cambridge: Cambridge University Press.

Walker, M. and van der Helm, E. (2009) 'Overnight therapy? The role of sleep in emotional brain processing'. *Psychological Bulletin*, 135 (5): 731–48.

Watson, C., Uberoi, E. and Kirk-Wade, E. (2022) *Women in Parliament and Government*. House of Commons Library. commonslibrary.parliament.uk.

Weinstein, Y. (2016) *Learn to Study Using ... Interleaving*. learningscientists.org.

Welch, N. (2021) *TransMidwife*. YouTube.

Wickham, S. (2006) *Appraising Research into Childbirth: An interactive workbook*. Edinburgh: Elsevier Butterworth-Heinemann.

Wickham, S. (2015) *101 Tips for Planning, Writing and Surviving your Dissertation*. UK: CreateSpace.

Wickham, S. (2017) *What is the BRAN Analysis?* sarawickham.com.

Wickham, S. (2018) *Pinard Wisdom (parts 1 and 2)*. https://www.sarawickham.com/articles-2/pinard-wisdom-part-1/; https://www.sarawickham.com/articles-2/pinard-wisdom-part-2/.

Wickham, S. (2019) *Cerridwyn and the Pixies: A Holiday Fairytale*. https://www.sarawickham.com/articles-2/cerridwyn-and-the-pixies-a-holiday-fairytale/.

Wickham, S. and Brown, A. (2022) *Another Study, Another Dodgy Headline! Please Don't Steal Our Coffee!* sarawickham.com.

Williams, K. (2021) Conversation with E. Durant [Interview].

Williams, M. (2020) *Oxford Uni Essay Writing Workshop!!* YouTube.

Winter, C., Crofts, J., Draycott, T. and Muchatuta, N. (2017) *PROMPT: Practical obstetric multi-professional training. Course manual*, 3rd edn. Cambridge: Cambridge University Press.

Women and Equalities Committee (2015) *Transgender Equality*. London: The Stationery Office.

Woolnough, H. and Fielden, S. (2017) *Mentoring in Nursing and Healthcare: Supporting career and personal development*. Chichester: Wiley Blackwell.

Xango, A. (2017) *Assetou Xango, Give Your Daughters Difficult Names*. Cafe Cultura, Denver. YouTube.

Yonis, A. (2018) *How to Get a 1st or 2:1 in ANY University Essay (with examples)*. YouTube.

Yonis, A. (2020) *Study Techniques to Avoid | Useless Revision Methods*. YouTube.

Yonis, A. (2021) *Top Study Methods for Visual Learners.* YouTube.

Young, A. (2021) 'How to remember what you learn for longer with spaced repetition'. blog.alexanderfyoung.com.

Young, H. (2020) Conversation with E. Durant [Interview].

Zwedberg, S., Alnervik, M. and Barimani, M. (2021) 'Student midwives' perception of peer learning during their clinical practice in an obstetric unit: a qualitative study'. *Nurse Education Today*, 99: 104785.

Index